Praise for *From Heart to Head & Back Again* ...

No industry depends more on engagement and on employees being connected to passion and purpose than healthcare. Knowing that you are making a difference in the lives of others is key to creating positive patient experiences and good clinical outcomes. The stories and reflections in these pages not only inspire us, they show us what real caring looks like in action. They show that even with the challenges our system faces, there are so many "flames of goodness" in healthcare. It's up to us as leaders to keep those flames burning bright. Thank you, Thomas, for this excellent book.

> Quint Studer
> Founder Studer Community Institute and Vibrant Community Partners
> Author of *A Culture of High Performance: Achieving Higher Quality at a Lower Cost; Hardwiring Excellence;* and many other highly impactful books.

Every so often you read a book that really makes you think. Also, every so often, you meet a person that really makes you think. It is a lucky and rare blessing to combine the two. Tom's book is one of those rare books that not only makes you think but also makes you feel.

I know Tom and consider him a friend. Tom is the kind of guy that when you spend five minutes with him you feel infinitely better about yourself. So how cool is it that he wrote a book? Now you can spend a few hours reading his book and walk away not only feeling better but being better.

You will walk away from this book knowing more, feeling more and wanting to be more. I can't recommend this book highly enough. We need a book like this these days.

I wish there were more people like Tom in this world.

Enjoy. Learn. Your heart will thank you.

> Rich Bluni, RN
> Senior Leader, Speaker, Author
> Author of *Inspired Nurse* & *Inspired Nurse Too*

Tom's book is troubling, inspiring, and thought-provoking all at the same time.

It's troubling to think that two experienced health care providers – Tom and his wife, Darlene – had such difficulty navigating the complexities of America's health care system.

It's inspiring because of their tremendous love for each other and their faith that sustained them through many difficult years trying to find help for Tom to the person he had been.

And it's thought-provoking to consider what role each of us can play – must play – to fix what's broken in our health care system.

It will take a new relationship between patient and physician, one of mutual respect, compassion, and commitment to healing. It's going to require a lot of conversations. Fortunately, in this book, Tom has already provided some of the important first questions to begin a dialogue.

> Kay Kendall
> CEO & Principal, Baldrige Coach
> Author of *Leading the Malcolm Baldrige Way: How World-Class Leaders Align Their Organizations to Deliver Exceptional Results*

Tom shares the story of his own healthcare experience, and how he navigated those months of care. He pours out his heart regarding the vulnerabilities he felt, even with the presence of a caring wife who is also a nurse. You can clearly feel the angst from his physical pain and worries brought forth from the emotional pain.

Tom reminds us that we can be the change we want to see in healthcare. His thought provoking stories serve as a checkpoint of how we are doing and where we need to be in terms of patient-centered care. It begs us to think of how we want those we serve and love to be cared for.

I would love to see this book utilized as an education tool for anyone in healthcare – physicians, nurses and ancillary staff that take part in touching patients' lives while helping them steer through the intricate world of healthcare. You will read this book and know that above all else, kindness and compassion matter in healthcare and in life.

> Jennifer Bowe, MSN, RN, RNC
> Clinical Director, Nursing
> Little Rock, AK

Tom shares the story of his compelling journey through our broken healthcare system, inspiring a call to action for those of us who want to make healthcare all about health and caring. I can think of no better person than Tom to inspire us to this great calling with a keen sense of urgency and compassion, connecting head and heart to truly make a difference in the lives of patients.

> Mark Hussey
> President & COO
> Huron

Through his courageous vulnerability and terrific storytelling, Tom successfully takes us on his journey through the healthcare system as both a patient and a leader, exposing flames of good within the system to be fanned and areas in which only together can we improve. His style is familiar (like an old friend), his insights brilliant, and his call to action one we all must heed. Join Tom on his journey and together let's improve the healthcare system for all.

> Jackie Gaines
> Senior Leader, Speaker, Author
> Author of *Believing You Can Fly*

From Heart to Head & Back Again ... a journey through the healthcare system is a provocative work that is part manifesto, part autobiography, and part manual. Tom offers us a transparent view into his transformative conversations with his quality improvement teams as a healthcare leader and moving conversations with his clinicians and wife as a critically ill patient. These diverse but synergistic perspectives offer us a glimpse into the "how to's" of building relationship-centered care that has the potential to reduce costs, boost outcomes, and transform our healthcare system from a place that too easily harms to a place that heals the heart, body, and spirit. This book includes reflection and discussion questions after every chapter and is "must read" for all healthcare professionals and leaders journeying to improve the quality of care of their patients and quality of life for themselves.

> Michelle Segar, PhD, MPH
> Director, University of Michigan's Sport, Health, and Activity Research and Policy Center
> Author of *No Sweat: How the Simple Science of Motivation Can Bring You a Lifetime of Fitness*

The tell-all book aptly titled *From Heart to Head & Back Again ...* is a peek into one man's healthcare journey that begs the reader to take part, to reflect, to ask and to answer questions as a way to improve today's healthcare system.

Whether you are a patient or a provider, Tom will cause you to join the 'troublemakers' to propel the movement to improve the patient experience.

A healthcare journey written from the perspective of both a healthcare leader and a patient whose passion for improving the system will ignite your desire to look inward and do the same.

>Pat Rullo
>Author, Speaker, Radio Host : Speak Up and Stay Alive Radio
>Podcast & Audiobook Narrator & Producer
>Author of *Highway to Heart, Humor, and Honesty in Healthcare*

Tom's book *From Heart to Head & Back Again - a journey through the healthcare system* is going to change the lives of every person in healthcare that is given the blessing of reading it. Tom is a part of the healthcare system. He knows the industry from the business perspective and also the caregiver perspective. The vulnerability he gently and passionately suggests to the reader will take them on a journey outside the bounds of our current healthcare system. This journey will cause each reader to create positive change to heal the collective brokenness of healthcare. It was an honor to be asked to read this book and it will be my honor to witness how it will affect the way we treat our caregivers, how they provide care: for themselves, their families, and us.

>Kristin Sunanta Walker
>CEO, MHNR Network
>Host, Mental Health News Radio
>CEO, everythingEHR: Behavioral Health Technology Solutions

From Heart to Head & Back Again ...

... a journey through the healthcare system

Thomas H. Dahlborg, Sr.

Copyright © 2020 DHLG

All rights reserved

Published by DHLG
Grand Rapids, MI 49546
Phone: 207-747-9663
https://tdahlborg.wordpress.com/
DahlborgHLG@gmail.com

ISBN-13: 9798646180736

The stories in this book are true. However, some names and identifying details have been changed to protect the privacy of all concerned.

All rights reserved. No part of this book may be used or reproduced in any form or by any means or stored in a database or retrieval system without the prior written permission of DHLG, except in the case of brief quotations embodied in critical articles or reviews. Making copies of any part of this book for any purpose other than your own personal use is a violation of United States copyright laws. Entering any of the contents into a computer for mailing list of database purposes is strictly prohibited unless written authorization is obtained from DHLG.

Printed in the United States of America.

Dedication

To my family. I love you.

To my amazing bride who is not only an incredible life partner to me and dedicated and loving mother to our children, but is also a brilliant and compassionate nurse who informs me daily of the reality of the front lines of healthcare, what it should be and how together we can make it so. I love you even more each day.

To my children. Each beautiful inside and out. Each full of passion and drive. Each teaching, leading and helping others. You are impacting, and that is what it is all about.

And to Gabriel, our papillon pup named for an angel, who role models unconditional love always.

To my parents, siblings and extended family who through a wide variety of lenses teach me daily.

To those on the front lines of healthcare. You hold great responsibility and touch many lives and souls. You are a blessing. Please take care of you as you take care of others.

To those leading, serving and loving in healthcare. The system needs you more now than ever. Thank you for showing up each day. Please take care of you too.

To all my teachers. Each of you. Thank you. You live on in my heart.

To all those who have been harmed by the healthcare system. We will do better.

To all those who have benefited from the healthcare system. We will do better.

To those who are discouraged. Please don't give up. And if you ever feel desperate, please seek help. We need you. We all need each other.

To all the *troublemakers* seeking to fix the brokenness within the system with courageous vulnerability. You are not alone. And if you ever feel that you are, please reach out. We are in this together.

And to the Ever-Living God, the Father – Son – Holy Spirit, thank you for blessing us all with Your majesty and ever-present Love.

Table of Contents

Foreword		18
Preface		19
Prologue	Brockton (1976)	23
Chapter 1	Prison (2001)	30
Chapter 2	A Broken Nose	33
Chapter 3	The Journey	35
Chapter 4	The First Day	40
Chapter 5	Missions and Mistakes	46
Chapter 6	Back at It	53
Chapter 7	Progress	62
Chapter 8	Taking on too much	70
Chapter 9	Voice of the Customer	79
Chapter 10	The Team	89
Chapter 11	Back to the VoC	97
Chapter 12	Mrs. Jones	102
Chapter 13	Voices of Our Customers	117
Chapter 14	Finding a Pathway to Honor our Patients	130
Chapter 15	The Flight	136
Chapter 16	Military Maneuvers	146
Chapter 17	Home from Seattle	154

Chapter 18	Back in the Office	159
Chapter 19	The Healthcare Alphabet	165
Chapter 20	Baseball and the Birthday Party (1997)	173
Chapter 21	Transport (1997)	185
Chapter 22	Shoulder Surgery (1997)	195
Chapter 23	Back to the Emergency Room (2001)	200
Chapter 24	Mercy Hospital	209
Chapter 25	For Everything	219
Chapter 26	The Couch	225
Chapter 27	Out of the Mouth of Babes	230
Chapter 28	The Birds	236
Chapter 29	The Visit	242
Chapter 30	Doctor's Orders	248
Chapter 31	The Robot	256
Chapter 32	The Call	263
Chapter 33	The Heart Attack	268
Chapter 34	Lose Me Forever	274
Chapter 35	Setting Records	280
Chapter 36	Blanket of Red	284
Chapter 37	Clean Shaven	292
Chapter 38	Unnecessary	298
Chapter 39	Surrender	306

Chapter 40	The Menu	313
Chapter 41	Resignation	319
Chapter 42	Goodbye	327
Chapter 43	A New Path	333
Chapter 44	Together	339
Chapter 45	Rest My Love	351
Chapter 46	A New Model	358
Chapter 47	A Second Chance	371
Chapter 48	Back to Work	379
Afterword		385
Acknowledgements		390
The Dove		394
Disruption		397

BONUS MATERIAL	399
The Gilded Age of Healthcare	400
Cultural Competence is a Leadership Choice – The Seven Steps	402
Hope Is Not A Strategy – It Is More Important	404
Author Bio	409

Foreword

The novel Coronavirus has shaken our society – and our health care system – to its core. But even as we mourn our losses and scramble to rise to new challenges, we are offered an opportunity: to take a hard look at the various levels of system dysfunction the pandemic exposes, and to choose to do better. For this, we need exemplars.

From Heart to Head & Back Again offers a much-needed, highly readable and enjoyable call to action: to double down on the human aspects of care that make patients feel known, understood, and cared for.

As Thomas Dahlborg points out:

> *Physicians pledge to honor the Hippocratic Oath, which includes the statement "... warmth, sympathy, and understanding may outweigh the surgeon's knife or the chemist's drug." Yet we do not create systems that allow for a focus on warmth and sympathy along with an appropriate balance of surgical, pharmaceutical, technological, and other medical / behavioral interventions.*

This speaks to the "dis-ease" that is plaguing our health care system: the price we've paid for clinical medicine's unswerving focus on empirically provable metrics, at the price of its propensity to dismiss as of lesser importance "what real people want". The fact that this has evolved from economic incentives makes it no less a failure in serving our humanity. While patients absolutely honor science (and appreciate that good clinical care is job #1), we deeply crave a system that's aligned with what we know in our gut (and what 1200 stories from patients and families shared with the Patients' View Institute affirm): as human beings, we value trust, accountability, respect and relationship above all. We never forget how people made us feel.

Focusing on respect, accountability and compassion will drive unknowable gains in safety, patient outcomes and clinician satisfaction, arising from a system in which everyone is positioned to thrive.

Dahlborg's book makes a personal, eloquent, and impassioned case for leaders to step up for this premise. For any organization looking to win the hearts and minds of patients in the 21st century, and to co-create a more functional, human-centric system of care, this book is a must-read.

Pat Mastors, President, Founder, Patients' View Partners
Former News Anchor / Medical Reporter, WPRI-TV

Preface

A few years back, the Deputy Commissioner of the State of Maine Department of Health & Human Services shared the administration's perspective on health policy in the state. She shared the goals of improving access, ensuring accountability, reducing costs and improving the health status of individuals and communities.

A question and answer session soon followed, along with a discussion concerning the challenges of emergency department (ED) overutilization.

A number of individuals stood up to impart how they were addressing the issue.

Solution plans shared included building hospital-owned urgent care centers closer to where high ED utilizers lived and building primary-care practices within the ED. Both would perhaps be effective and definitely costly.

And then it happened ... before I could look up and share my thoughts, a physician assistant (PA) from Northern Maine was selected to speak and shared the following:

> *"I know how to address the issue of overutilization of emergency departments. I do it every day. I know the people who would utilize the ED. I talk to these people and I listen to these people. I have developed relationships with these people. They know me and I know them. We trust one another. When they have a concern, they call me and we talk. And when they should come to the ED they do. And when there are better options, I help them to understand those options. It is all about relationship and trust."*

This PA on a daily basis lives what many "experts" can only surmise. This amazing individual is in a system where she positively impacts the lives of patients and families, saves the system money, and is doing so by leveraging relationship. Relationship. Empathy. Trust. And the ability to truly listen and understand.

How amazing and wonderful and inexpensive and effective and a "no brainer." Right? Perhaps not...

I went up to this PA (who I had met a few months prior) hugged her and said how much I appreciated what she said. She in turn told me that she was surprised they selected her to speak as she is considered a troublemaker in her organization.

A troublemaker?

> Well ... "Here's to the crazy ones. The misfits. The rebels. The troublemakers. The round pegs in the square hole. The ones who see things differently. They're not fond of rules. And they have no respect for the status quo. You can quote them, disagree with them, glorify or vilify them. About the only thing you can't do is ignore them. Because they change things. They push the human race forward. And while some may see them as the crazy ones, we see genius. Because the people who are crazy enough to think they can change the world, are the ones who do." – Apple Computer, Inc.

I left that Q&A session having been reminded of two important lessons. First, listen and heed the input from the so-called "troublemakers" (who in many cases are people on the front lines of healthcare). They are the ones in the know. And as Apple recognizes, "They will push us all forward. They will change the world."

Second, ensure that relationship, empathy, trust and the ability to truly listen become as important to the healthcare model, as any new alternative payment model, any new revenue generation strategy, any new technological advancement, or any other "innovation".

Thank you, my Physician Assistant friend, for saying so beautifully what we all needed to hear. And thank you for the perfect beginning to this book.

This book is a journey.

A journey which has blessed me with the ability and desire to now listen and embrace the message of the "troublemakers", like the PA in Northern Maine who courageously each day is making things better for others.

A journey which has both humbled me and educated me so that I too can open my head (my mind) and heart in order to better lead and serve.

A journey of learning courage through vulnerability. Of learning that it is not a sign of weakness to care (especially for a male in our society). Of learning that there is great goodness within the healthcare system and opportunities to make a difference. And that only together can we do so.

Join me and together let's improve the healthcare system for our patients and families, our doctors and nurses, for all the healthcare workers and for our communities.

Prologue

Brockton (1976)

The shade from the oaks and pines were clouding first and second base. My shadow extended well past the pitcher. My shadow even taller and thinner than me.

"Invisible men on second and third."

"No there isn't! There is no invisible man at third," came back the response from my best friend Mitchell.

Mitchell was a year younger than me. A good-looking kid with brown hair and an easy smile. Always something up his sleeve. Always seeking an advantage. An edge. An extra cookie or a swim in a neighbor's pool. Yes. My best friend.

"Yes, there is!"

And for the next few moments I explained in fine detail to Mitchell and his older brother Barry why there was and how they got there.

Barry was my older brother Jon's age, 13. While Jon typically won't play sports with me, Barry on occasion makes an appearance. He is far more passionate about Scouts than sports, but on this sunny August day with the chance to team up with his little brother and beat me he was on the field of play.

"Whatever."

Yes! Mitchell knew I was right. I always knew the score, the inning, what was happening on the field, what just happened, and what must be done to be successful … to win.

You must growing up in Brockton, Massachusetts, home of two of the greatest boxers in history.

Or I should say "I must" growing up in this city. No sacrifice is too much. Pain is a badge of honor. Be "Brockton-tough" I learned.

Rocky Marciano is the only heavyweight champion with a perfect record (49 wins in 49 professional bouts). Of these wins, 43 were knockouts. No other fighter fought like he did. Smaller than many of his opponents. He was known for his toughness. His tenacity. He took on all comers. He gave no quarter. And he always won.

And by the time of this kickball game in mid-August of 1976, Marvelous Marvin Hagler had already rung up a record of 28 wins (22 by knockout or TKO), 2 losses, and 1 draw and by the end of the year would become the Middleweight Champion of the World.

Brockton itself also had a reputation … as a blue-collar city. During the Civil War and up until the latter parts of the 20th Century, Brockton was known as America's largest producer of shoes and, in fact, by the turn of the century there were over 91 shoe factories in the city. People worked hard and were known to be physically and mentally strong.

Yes, a lot to live up too. Work hard. Be tough. Give no quarter. And WIN.

So here we were. We had agreement (kind of) that there were two outs in the bottom of the last inning. I was losing 11 to 9. There were two invisible men on base, one of these on second and the other on third … and Mitchell was on the mound ready to pitch.

The sun was shining over my shoulder as sweat dripped down my now pink neck and under my white t-shirt.

My breath was shallow and quick as the thought of potentially losing this game weighed heavily on my mind.

I note the sun in Mitchell's eyes as he struggles to see me at home plate. I see Barry standing in right field under the shade of a tree squinting to see the action before him.

And I note a gap in deep left field.

Mitchell readies and rolls the ball toward home plate.

I got this.

I feel my foot make less than solid contact on the ball and yet as I look up, I see the ball traveling in a line toward the gap.

Yes!

I sprint toward first base and as I am running, I hear Mitchell call out, "Barry, get the ball. I'll take the cut!"

As I round first base and head toward second, I am surprised that Barry has not yet emerged with the ball.

Apparently, Mitchell was too, "Barry! Hurry!!"

I reach second and still no Barry.

Breathing heavily, I continue my sprint and am now headed for third as Mitchell heads toward the flat rock we call home plate.

As I reach third, I see that Barry is still deep in left so I decide to round the base and go for the win.

As I turn toward home all I see is Mitchell's body illuminated from behind by the sun which is now directly behind his head and shining into my eyes.

Through the haze of the late August sun, I see Mitchell catch Barry's throw at chest level as I charge toward this Fisk-ian pitcher turned catcher.

I also see through the haze and shadow the ferocity in which Mitchell is about to launch this sphere at my head. (Kickball in Brockton is clearly not for the faint of heart.) And his snarl as his eyes crocodile, and he whips his right arm forward and unloads.

But just as Hagler would slip past a Sugar Ray left jab, I make my move and …

The joy of winning was short.

Ugh. I am in trouble again.

We live in a ranch house on the south side of Brockton. The west side is the rich side.

My father is a schoolteacher. He teaches science at West Junior High School. There he teaches 7th and 8th graders and develops a reputation as a hard ass. His "sludge test" final has already created many a nervous breakdown for kids. But overall, he is well liked and respected.

My mother is an x-ray technician by training and works as a Title I teacher's aide. She is an amazing budgeter and keeps the family afloat with her financial prowess.

My brother is a far better athlete than I, but sports are truly not his passion. Be it baseball, tennis, basketball, hockey, he can do them all well and seemingly without much effort. "Naturally gifted Jon is," my father would say. And yet, Jon prefers Sci-Fi movies to baseball by a long shot.

Me? Sports are my life. School? Books? Movies? Nope. All I want to do is use my body, feel exertion, and feel the ache of victory (even in a loss) that comes when you have done everything possible in order to win. That is all I want. All I ever want. Each night I think about Dwight

Evans' amazing catch in right field against the Reds in the 1975 World Series, the Bruins' Brad Park dishing out hard hip-checks against all daring to enter his space, Dave Cowens' ferocity under the boards as he leads the Celtics to their most recent championship, and most of all, my hero, Roger Staubach leading comebacks with determination and guts for my Dallas Cowboys. And each day I wake with this unnamed desire always just below the surface of my reality waiting for the moment when we say … GAME ON!

Yes. Sports. And yes, I will be in big trouble when I get home.

As I stand, I feel an ache in my right knee.

Yes, the ache of victory.

But then an old reality kicks in. I know this ache.

Since I was very little, I have had pain in both my knees. Pain that feels like someone or something has bored a hole from the inside of my right knee clear through to the other side. Pain that feels like someone has slammed the side of my left knee over and over again with a sledgehammer. An intense ache that finds no relief and little sympathy. A pain I have both suffered through and used as a motivator to push my body further than it was designed to be pushed.

But even prior to these pains, when I was very young, the doctor prescribed that I wear leg braces, which as I recall consisted of leather shoes attached to a metal contraption with a steel bar connecting my left foot to my right.

Each night my parents would say to me, "Tommy, it is time to put on your 'cowboy boots,'" and I would crawl over to have this apparatus bound to me and then crawl back to my toys or books dragging my legs and this steel prison behind me.

And each morning I would wake early and climb over my bed rails with my leg shackles in tow. All the while thinking, *Please mom, please, take my cowboy boots off.*

Yes, each night I would have my cowboy boots put on and each morning they would be removed. Day after day and night after night. Until the day when I was released from this torture, able to move my legs freely, and finally slumbered through an entire evening.

Now, years later when my legs are hurting, I think back to my "cowboy boots" and to the many doctors who told my mom, "There is nothing wrong with your son's knees. You simply have an active child who needs to be more careful."

And here in August of 1976 in the aftermath of the kickball game to end all kickball games …

I can't go home and tell my parents I hurt my knee. I just can't. We cannot afford it, and more importantly, ... they will tell me to stop playing.

REFLECTION

Over the years I made note of how interesting it was that folks in Brockton decide who you are and what you will become simply based on the side of town you live on. Want to be a doctor? Make sure you live on the west side.

I also learned to not make assumptions about people based on where they live, their color, their creed, their socio-economic standing, religion, and so much more.

It is far more important to share time and truly get to know someone than to jump to any conclusions based on an assumption or an average person.

Years later I would see this play out in medical research and other aspects of healthcare as research based on an "average" person (which does not exist) was extrapolated to apply to all people and "cookie cutter" standards of care were applied with no clear understanding that each patient is unique, a complex adaptive system, and thus an "average" approach was not optimal for anyone.

Questions

1. As a healthcare leader, clinician, staff person, patient or family member, how has your childhood shaped you?
    a. How do assumptions help or hinder you within the healthcare system?
2. As a healthcare leader, clinician, or staff person, tell a story of a time when you made an assumption about a patient or family in healthcare and the impact.
    a. What did you learn?
    b. How have you mitigated any predilection to making assumptions about patients and families?

Chapter 1

Prison (2001)

A faint calling. Barely audible and yet slowly and patiently growing louder.

The grey walls are moving again. Violently tossed aside with a determined ferocity as the vice across my chest grabs hold.

"Is that you Mare of the Vettes pouncing on my chest and eliciting this mardröm?"

Nightmares are not new to me. "Bring it on," I want to scream ... but this is different.

"Frazier!" I hear Howard Cosell bellow. "Frazier!"

But this time, Frazier is not going down.

"Ali's jaw is broken. Frazier broke Ali's jaw!"

No. It's not Ali's jaw. It is my jaw. Frazier hit me with the right cross.

"Frazier broke my jaw!"

Thoughts and sounds are becoming one. "Am I awake? Is this real?!"

From behind me, I feel someone grasp my face.

"They are strangling me!"

"You are strangling me!" I scream in my head as I am being smothered. "I can't breathe!"

And then the Stabbing. "Et tu, Brute?"

"Cut him! Cut him!"

"I am going to die!" I scream as I see my family float into sight ... My bride, the love of my life; Samantha, my beautiful seven-year-old first born; Tommy, my rambunctious five-year-old; Haylee, my three-year-old porcelain doll; and Angus, my beloved pup.

"I love you. I love you. My God, I love you all so."

The cuts are glancing blows.

The first to the right side of my chest.

The second in the same area but on the left side.

Another just below the second cut.

Then at the fourth in the 'fifth intercostal space at the midclavicular line'.

I'm losing track now.

I feel a pulling near my ankle.

And then a pressure between my elbow and shoulder.

"I'm cut!"

I'm bleeding now from my left arm.

I need to move. "Get up, Tom. Run!" I demand.

"IV fluids are all set."

"Run it, KVO!"

"Yes, doctor!"

"Good. Finish setting the 12-lead and have the ECG to me stat."

"Yes, doctor."

"Doctor? Who is hurt and why are they in my prison cell?" I demand of the Universe.

It's cold again. I feel an intense chill flowing up my left arm and into my shoulder and chest.

"Tom."

I hear my name being called through the denseness of my cell.

"Tom. My name is Carol. You are in the Emergency Room at Mercy Hospital. Your friend brought you here. You have an IV in your left arm providing you with fluids. You have a mask over your nose and mouth. Just continue to breathe normally. We are giving you oxygen to help with your breathing. I am now hooking you up to the ECG machine to monitor your heart rhythm. Do you understand me?"

Mercy Hospital. I am at Mercy.

"Phlebotomy will be in shortly to draw blood."

"Okay. But for what?" I hear echo off the walls of my prison.

"We want to rule out that you are having a heart attack."

"A heart attack? I am only 35-years-old."

Chapter 2

A Broken Nose

The arctic air within this solitude is freezing my whole as my body tremors in spite of my will. And yet this is not Camp Barneo, and I am not a Russian scientist.

The greyness of my surroundings is not new (being color blind makes it the norm), but why is it so cold and why are my walls moving? If Boreas has chosen this day to venture into my space and whip up these cold winds for my entertainment, I would just as soon Zeus act the lead deity in this play and tell the Anemoi, "Be gone, and leave this mortal be."

And the brightness emanating from upon high? I squint as I look up toward heaven in hopes of finding salvation as the sun blasts its rays upon my face and yet without their customary warmth.

What is that? I say to myself as I focus on the discordance between temperature and light.

A noise. No. A beep. A beeping below the surface of consciousness ... or is it? I say as the cacophony of sound bellows in my ears.

More noise. *A child. A child is crying*, I think, as additional noises begin to flood my surroundings. *Sammy! Tommy! Haylee! Where are MY children?*

"Tom. I am here. Oh honey, I am here. What happened? Your office called me and said you were in the hospital. What happened?!" Darlene (aka Doc), my bride, whispers to me from a beach to this soul lost at sea.

My wife is here. I am saved, my mind begins to repeat as one of the walls holding me prisoner for so long is ripped open and a tall guard, perhaps the warden, with deep set black eyes, dark hair, and a white coat enters and stares down at me.

"You can't breathe!? I know why you can't breathe," is shot at me like the sound of an M-16. "You have a broken nose!"

And then she was gone.

"A broken nose? I was with Maureen looking at houses when your office called. They said you were in the hospital. Maureen has the kids. Tom, what happened?"

Chapter 3

The Journey

The healthcare system is profoundly broken. Each day we are harming our doctors and nurses, our patients and families, our communities, and one another.

Symptoms of this brokenness are evident when we hear, "We cannot do the right thing until the financial drivers change."

And, "I don't have time for quality. My job is to increase the hospital's market share."

And when we see the percent of preventable adverse events that take place for each and every hospital admission.

We can do better. We must.

And yet there are great people sacrificing themselves inside and outside of the system daily in order to make a difference and positively impact the life of another.

This book is a call to action. It serves to bring together these people (each of you, each of us), who truly have the wisdom, the character, the energy, the passion, and the heart, to make a difference, to do what is right, to lead and to serve, and to make a positive impact for others.

For a number of years' people have asked me to write "my story." A story from the perspective of both a healthcare leader and a patient.

And each time I heard this message I said, "No. My story isn't worthy. There are far better, more worthy and more impactful stories."

And yet, with the encouragement of my wife and family, friends and colleagues, and many others, I embarked on this story-telling journey. Yes, battling my own instincts to share "my story."

> Questions:
>
> Have you ever gone through a significant experience, be it health related or other, and by the time it was over all you wanted to do was forget all about it?
>
> Just think about that for a moment. Perhaps you were told your child was very ill. You and your significant other mourn the news at first … but then what? You go into action mode. Yes. Just like the first question many of us ask of another when we first meet, "What do you do?" We are an action society. We *do*.
>
> So, you learn that your child, or parent, or spouse, or friend, or self are very ill. You go into action mode. You make things happen. There are times when you fight the system, and there are times when the system fights you. But lo and behold, at some point you come out the other end. The specific crisis is over. Ideally with a happy ending. Sometimes not.
>
> But then what?
>
> How many of us reflect on that journey? How many of us assess our own wellbeing, the lessons learned, our growth, our good decisions, our poor decisions, our decisions that may have led to harm to another? Or how many of us simply say "Glad that is over!" And, "I hope I never have to go through that again!"

That said, reading this book and joining me on this journey is meant to be an interactive experience that includes processing, assessing, reflecting, acknowledging, responding, and ideally when we do our jobs right, the creation of a movement.

Yes. I said it. A movement. A movement where together, collaboratively, we learn and share with one another. We leverage our wonderfully varied lenses and share stories, some incredibly powerful and moving and others not, and yet all important because they are OUR stories.

I seek the input of the patient and family, the nurse and the doctor, the hospital CEO and the phlebotomist. I seek information from the insurance executive, the physician practice administrator, the patient advocate, the front desk clerk, the ambulance driver, and the nursing home administrator. In short, I seek wisdom from all of you who have engaged the healthcare system and seek change.

And I ask that as you read this book, you be mindful of which hat you are wearing at any given time and that when you share, you acknowledge that you are seeing through the lens of a nurse, or a doctor, or a family member, or a patient, etc. as you do so.

I ask that you open your hearts and minds as you read and as you share and maintain a focus on improving the system for all.

I ask that you acknowledge that when my story, and the stories within the story, trigger you, that you share your thoughts, add additional insights and perspectives, and be bold and courageous as you do, so that we can learn and grow together and save the lives of those we are currently harming.

For example, when I write of an amazing person within the healthcare system who helped me greatly, perhaps you have a similar story you would like to share, or perhaps you have a story that reflects an opposite experience. Please share.

And if you are prompted by another aspect of my story, perhaps a bad experience I highlight, and yet you have sat on the other side of the table and can empathize with another point of view and/or shed light on a new or different perspective ... I ask you to again share so we can all learn and grow.

Perhaps you are a physician who understands what it is like each day to try to find a way to share with a family that their beloved mother has passed away ... and to do so professionally, with respect, and dignity, and love. And then ten minutes later, you must greet a new patient, someone completely new to you whose medical record you have not had time to review, all while being quite aware you are booked back-to-back for the remainder of the day, have a stack of paperwork to complete and boxes to click before you can even find a moment to check in with yourself to ensure you are okay after having delivered such hard news to the family with compassion.

Please share.

Perhaps you are a hospital CFO and above all else, you want to ensure your hospital remains financially viable in order to provide access to quality care in the community. I ask you as well to reflect, to share your perspective, and to help us fix the system.

Or a healthcare insurance executive, a patient account representative, a daughter of an amazing women who has loved and cared for you all your life and who is now on her dying journey, the husband of a young wife with three children who is dying of cancer, a coach who has seen far too many female athletes suffer from torn ACLs, and more.

We need all of these insights.

Perhaps you yourself are facing the daily challenges of managing a chronic illness. Please share your story.

As you have read in the prologue to this book and its first couple of chapters, I am exposing my vulnerability to all of you.

I ask you to also be vulnerable. And to share bravely in order to help us make a difference.

Yes, courage and healing through vulnerability.

Where did you fail? (Please think of it as failing forward as a friend of mine would say). What did you learn? How can we leverage these learnings to do better?

The same holds true for successes of course. Please share.

I am sure you have also noted by now that I have shared some of my upbringing as part of this story. Yes. To both provide context but also to acknowledge that each of our upbringings, our backgrounds, our life experiences, and so much more have shaped our thinking, our lives. Here I ask you to be mindful of the impact of our backgrounds, and the shadows we bear and the projections we make onto others, and to again be open with both our hearts and minds as we read, reflect and respond, and continue on this improvement and innovation pathway together.

So yes, I ask you to share. I ask you to be vulnerable. I ask you to be brave. I ask you to be mindful. And most of all, I ask you to help us all identify what is truth within the system and how together we can fix it.

This book is just the beginning.

The healthcare system that I (and many of you) have helped to create is doing great good.

And the healthcare system that I (and many of you) have helped to create is also doing great harm to those we cherish.

Those we are harming need us.

"But how are we going to make a difference?"

"But how are we going to share?"

At the end of many sections of this book you will find one or more of the following:
1. My own reflections for you to consider
2. Questions for you to consider and respond to

And when or if you do decide to share your reflections, insights, wisdom, your story, or ask a question, here is my E-mail and my cell phone number (I want to hear from you) …

DahlborgHLG@gmail.com
207-747-9663

… and together we will write the next healthcare chapter.

This book is not about shame and blame; that doesn't work with what the system calls 'non-compliant patients,' and it won't work to improve the healthcare system.

This book is about a movement that involves you. A movement to honor one another, each of our stories, and make the system better … for all.

This book is based on my work as a healthcare leader (who has worked within the healthcare system for the past thirty-five years) and as a patient who nineteen years ago was told he would never work again.

Each vignette highlights either a flame of goodness within the system that we must continue to fan, a challenge that together we must overcome, or an experience which will perhaps call to mind a similar experience for you and, as noted, allow for your own personal reflection (which may be 180 degrees opposite of mine) and sharing …and perhaps your own healing.

Margaret (Meg) Wheatley recently shared much that aligns greatly with what I also espouse, e.g., the importance of building strong relationships, the importance of collaboration in addressing challenges, and the essential need for personal reflection.

(NOTE: These are also essential for our journey together.)

She also shared that she does not believe we can change the system.

I hope she is wrong. Because of people like you, I still believe. I still have hope. And yes, hope is not a strategy … it is actually more important. Hope is the foundation for all.

So, let's journey through this story together, let's share our own stories, let's identify those places where we each can make our own personal changes, where together we can improve aspects of the health and healthcare system, and where in relationship and with trust, our service to others will have the biggest impact for our patients, our families, our communities and for one another.

Let's share these insights and wisdom and together let's write the next story that honors each of YOUR stories, shares our collective wisdom and recommendations to improve the system, and highlights what a group of people with a similar mission and working together can do to improve this world.

Together we will make a difference.

Chapter 4

The First Day

I had recently accepted a leadership role with a military healthcare organization in Maine. And on this early morn in December of 1999 I was heading North ahead of my family to begin the next phase of my career.

It was a bitterly cold morning when I packed the trunk of my silver Jetta with the Christmas light dashboard, kissed my three beautiful sleeping children on their foreheads, patted my pup, and hugged my loving wife.

We had been married seven years at this point and on numerous occasions over that time period, Doc had nursed me back to health. Yes, I was very strategic in marrying a nurse.

We had fallen in love quickly and remained in love … even as I was pulling her away from her friends and family for this new opportunity. My new mission.

And I was so grateful for her and our forever partnership.

That morning as I reached the Piscataqua Bridge connecting New Hampshire and Maine, I remember thinking about my three children, Sammy who would be six in January, Tommy who was almost exactly three and a half years old, and Haylee who just had her first birthday in November. They were getting so big.

As I passed a Biddeford Exit, I continued to process. This time about my pup, Angus. Such a good pup who came into our lives after we had lost Chewbacca, who had lived with epilepsy and a debilitating skin condition for so many years (and who, by the way, encouraged Doc to fall in love with me in the first place).

As Doc tells it, she was still assessing me. Was I "the one"? Was I worthy of her love? And then one day we walked into my parent's kitchen and she saw a ball of matted, oily, slimy fur jump out from under an antique cabinet and come limping over toward us. Disgusted at first at the sight and smell she recalled, "When I saw this thing heading our way, I was quite repulsed. But then I saw you get down on your hands and knees and love this creature without hesitation. That was when I saw your heart. That was when I knew you would be a good father to my children. That is when I knew I loved you."

"Thank you, Chewbacca. I love and miss you."

As I reached Kennebunk, I knew it was time to call my bride.

"Doc, I am in Kennebunk. I miss you already."

"I miss you too. The kids are still sleeping but I am up drinking a cup of Dunks while sitting on the couch watching the sun rise. How is your head? How is your shoulder?"

"I can feel my shoulder and there is some pain shooting through my neck and into my head, but I am fine."

"I am sorry dear. Don't forget to take your Naproxen this morning … and be sure to do so with food."

By 8:15am, I pulled into the parking lot and mentally prepared to go in and meet with my new team.

By 8:25am, I walked through the door.

"Tom! We have been waiting for you. Well, not literally. Well, actually literally. Oh, never mind. What I mean is we are thrilled you are here."

It was Lisa, the HR Director who recruited me … now for the second time.

My office was nice with a solid dark brown desk, a comfy ergonomically correct chair, a bookshelf and a credenza, and a small round table with two chairs for one on one discussions. All it was missing was a picture of my bride in her wedding gown, taken the morning of our wedding by her father, a Christmas picture of our three children taken just a week ago at Sears, and of course a picture of Angus with the tan heart on his side.

"There," I said after carefully placing each picture and taking a moment to hold them close to my heart even with me a hundred and fifty miles away.

"It looks like you are settling in very well. I love your family pictures."

"Very much so, Lisa. Thank you."

"So let me walk you down to the Network Development quad and reintroduce you to your team."

"James, Jesse, Debbie, Denise … I would like to re-introduce you to Tom. Tom, here is your team."

"It is so wonderful to be here, team. When we met a few weeks back and you each shared your vision for this department, along with your challenges and concerns, I knew I wanted to work with you. And clearly we have much to do together and that begins with us determining … where we are going to lunch?"

Over lunch and throughout the day I learned a great deal more about my team.

I learned that James is ex-Navy. (Hence, the strong handshake.) He is also the leader of the group (clearly) which I noted during the group interview. He has a deep voice, penetrating eyes, and cares deeply about doing a good job. Leader is the word that is apparent for James.

Jesse is a young dad. He is tall with brown hair parted to the side. Handsome and clean cut. He is extremely bright, which is also extremely obvious and just as obvious is the fact he doesn't realize how bright he is. Jesse is also very conscientious and caring and best of all (just kidding … kind of) a basketball fan. Earnest is the word that jumps out to me for Jesse.

Debbie comes across less secure about herself and her role. And yet, her passion for her team, for the organization, and her eagerness to learn and grow and contribute are very conspicuous. When I think of Debbie, the word teammate comes straight to mind.

And Denise appears a bit younger than the rest of the team. I learned that while each of the others is actively engaging directly with external providers, she is focused on the administrative aspects of the department including the provider directory.

As a team, I also picked up the fact that there is great energy, smarts, passion, and heart here. What was lacking previously was clear direction from up on high, solid leadership beyond the team, and trust of the team. This team was a captain-less ship, and now I believed I could help them.

Later that evening I called Doc, "Yes, I can provide value here. These people are amazing. They care. That is what I want. That is what I wanted. Give me people who care and are passionate, and we will change the world. I will first listen and then, with their insights and wisdom, I will teach and coach them the rest of the way."

"Oh Tom …"

"Doc, all they need is a leader who understands, who cares, and who will break down barriers and ensure a clear mission and understood strategy. I am so excited!"

"… you are truly meant to be there. And we are meant to be there in Maine with you."

REFLECTION

In quality improvement-speak, we often ask: What can you do by next Tuesday to make a difference?

Here, I will change this just a bit.

I will ask: Who will you listen to right now to make a difference?

Recently, I was speaking with a patient safety advocate from Sweden who was sharing much about her organization along with both the flames of goodness within the Swedish healthcare system and the areas for improvement. The discussion was amazing, as was the mutual learning.

But it was one specific thing she said that truly caught my attention more than anything else:

> "Tom, there was so much energy and passion for ensuring our patients are safe. In fact, when I began my organization the number of people from throughout the healthcare system willing to donate time and energy was overwhelming. But soon, the sad reality set in for them ... as it did for me. Almost every one of these energized, smart, caring people quickly realized that if they were to continue to focus on patient safety, they would lose their jobs within the system. Oh tom, so sad and yet so true. What a loss at so many levels. Why don't these individuals' respective leaders listen to understand how this work not only improves patient safety for all but also enhances their staff's passions and refuels these people to contribute even more so in their everyday roles?"

This past week, I was checking in with an incredible person, a cardiologist who continues to brave her own health challenges as she also seeks to find a place within the healthcare system where she can lead, serve, and make a difference. She shared:

> "I'm so disheartened and feel I need help imagining how I can go forth."

And during my monthly internet radio healthcare segment, a passionate visiting nurse shared with me:

> "I can't tell you the number of scales that I have purchased over my career for people [who could not afford one on their own] just to help them maintain and monitor their weight–because that is the no. 1 step in managing congestive heart failure."

She also highlighted many of the adverse impacts to both patients and the system of simply not providing to a patient a scale in which to monitor his or her weight, including the costs associated with readmissions and treatment protocols.

She also emphatically asked:

> "When we have someone in a wheelchair, why are we not giving them a $100 roho cushion to prevent the bedsores? Why not give it to them before we have two stage 2 bedsores, which require that I go out there three times per week?"

She went on to share additional insights into prevention opportunities that improve patient care, improve patient experience, lower costs, and prevent readmissions.

And as she did, she also shared her frustration that those in healthcare leadership positions are not listening to nurses and others on the front lines who have insights that can inform their decision-making and ultimately lead to significant improvements in care and outcomes.

These are just three examples of smart, caring people seeking to improve safety, to get back into action, to improve care, to reduce costs, and to make things better.

And in each case, they are seeking someone within the system to listen to them, to care about them and their mission, to ensure they and their teams are safe ... and to truly understand.

Questions

1. As a healthcare leader, clinician, staff person, patient or family member, who will you listen to right now to make a difference?
2. As a clinician or staff person, who needs to hear your insights and how will you ensure they do?
3. As a patient or family member, within the healthcare system, are you truly listened to relative to your insights and wisdom?
4. What would you recommend to ensure the nuggets of wisdom from throughout the healthcare system are not lost but rather truly listened to, honored, and used to improve care for us all?

Chapter 5

Missions and Mistakes

Later that evening as I thought more about my first day, I realized that not only did we have big hills to climb but also ... I had screwed up.

Yes, the mission of the organization touched my heart, my mind, my soul ... 'to exemplify and inspire healthcare and service excellence through leadership, education and innovation.' And yes, the challenges before me and my team were striking.

There were thousands of military dependents and military retirees who did not have appropriate access to care. The system was placing them in harm's way because our commitment to them had not been honored. (Not due to lack of trying. But, from my perspective, rather due to a lack of focus and leadership.) Our members were not accessing the right care at the right time in the right location and thus were not only not receiving good healthcare ... they were being harmed.

This organization had big challenges, and I desperately wanted to lead and serve with my team to meet them. But perhaps I was too eager to show just that.

Throughout the recruitment process I had learned that I would be working side by side with a number of ex-military personnel who cared deeply about their brethren and were essentially internal advocates for each and every one of them.

Walking in that first day I believed that the wisdom I had garnered over the previous fifteen years working within the healthcare system would help me to address many of the challenges before me while also fanning the flames of what was already working. I believed that through my heart, I would embrace this mission and the values of the organization and both serve and lead my team while focusing their energy on those critical few things within our control that would have the biggest impact. And I believed my soul (my love) would encompass it all.

But I screwed up.

Throughout that first day, I realized more and more that the strong pull I had for this organization and its mission to be of service to those who have served this country and their families could not compare (not even in the least) with the connection people such as our military folk have for their compatriots.

When I met with Stephen earlier that day, I learned that he became a member representative for us in order to ensure that military families and retirees were made aware of all the benefits available to them (including our program), and when or if they found our program best that they were well positioned to join.

I recall sitting in his cubicle and seeing on his face the responsibility he felt for ensuring his brothers and sisters in arms were being appropriately cared for. I also recall seeing from his body position that as I shared my passion for this very same mission that perhaps I came across as 'salesy' rather than authentic.

Stephen had been here long enough to see that the organization was not honoring its commitment to our members (and potential members). And here I was the "new guy" from Boston with no military background saying how important this was to me and how we were going to fix this with absolutely no credibility in the eyes of someone who had truly served.

No doubt he had heard all I had to say previously ... and up to this point it was all just words.

I also reflected back on my meeting with James that first day. And noted that even longer than Stephen he had lived with the fact that to date the organization had not honored its mission to the military families.

And then there was Esther. Esther Newbury was already an amazing woman in my eyes. Throughout the recruitment process, many had shared much of Esther's background ... 22 years' active duty Navy, 9 years enlisted Hospital Corpsman, and 13 years commissioned Medical Service Corps Officer. And how the previous year she was brought here to administer our huge contract with the Department of Defense for this military healthcare program.

But even all this prep work did not prepare me for Esther.

Thinking back to our meeting earlier that afternoon:

"Hi Esther. I am Tom. The new Director of Provider Networks."

"I know who you are. I am unclear as to why I was not asked to interview all the candidates for that role. Ensuring our members (the military dependents and retirees, not the active duty personnel I will remind you) have access to care is a DoD requirement. We have not met this requirement in the past and I am not intending to inform the government that we have not met this requirement again. Do you understand?"

"I understand, Esther."

But did I really?

"My goal is to honor that mission. My goal is to ensure my team provides adequate access..."

"Adequate? Your goal is to be adequate?"

Darn it!

I said that term because when building networks of physicians and hospitals the managed healthcare term used to measure access is "network adequacy." I should have thought more before speaking and using such jargon. Especially with someone who is clearly so passionate. Clearly being "adequate" is not good enough for those who have given so much. And it cannot be good enough for us.

I tried again.

"My goal is to ensure we meet the DoD access standards and then, once met, to exceed those standards with only the highest quality physicians we can credential."

"Be sure that you do."

At the time of our discussion, I remember thinking how tough Esther was. As I processed more later that evening things changed ...

Esther is military. Esther knows honor. Esther cares deeply about the military families. She is well aware that our organization has not honored its mission. She was also excluded from the process to hire for a key position, which is greatly responsible for improving access for these people. And this "business guy" who she did not hire used the term adequate (which can mean "barely sufficient") when discussing plans to try to improve the care for these military folks.

And it was at this time I pledged ...

This is not just a job for these people. And this "mission" is clearly far beyond the mission of other for-profits, and not-for-profits for that matter, I have served. Yes, I am passionate about this mission. Yes, I am here because of this mission. Yes, I am going to do all I can to achieve this mission. And yes, I cannot truly understand what Stephen, James, and Esther feel each day knowing that we let their brothers and sisters down.

REFLECTION

I recently had the opportunity to speak with a brilliant physician and chief experience officer (who I will refer to as Dr. Jane Sloan) at a large healthcare institution with reach and impact both nationally and internationally.

It did not take long for Dr. Sloan and me to realize we shared not only many philosophies and a vision for healthCARING, but also a common language.

Many folks talk of patient experience, patient engagement, and patient activation, but Dr. Sloan and I homed in on our shared focus on "relationship-centered care" and the importance of:

- *Each member of the care team developing authentic relationships with their patients and families*

- *Healthcare leaders developing care models (healthCARING models) that position the care team, i.e., physicians, nurses, physician assistants, etc., to be whole and healthy themselves*

- *Using structures, learnings, processes and financial drivers to enhance the relationship between care team and patient and family, rather than to create barriers.*

Together we also noted that patient-centered care in and of itself is not enough.

One explanation of relationship-centered care (RCC) comes from Mary Catherine Beach, M.D., Thomas Inui, M.D., and the Relationship-Centered Care Research Network:

> "Relationship-centered care is health enhancing. It is founded upon, proceeds within and is significantly influenced by the web of relationships that promote the well-being and full functioning of patients. In RCC, the patient is often our central concern, but is not considered in isolation from all others. Instead, while the clinicians' first responsibility is to prevent and alleviate illness, we do this work mindful of the contributions of the family, our team, our organizations and our community to what can be accomplished. Similarly, we must be mindful of the impact of what we do with patients on the well-being of all others involved, including their integrity, functional capacity, resilience and financial stability. Finally, we do this work in full knowledge that our own

well-being and function need to be sustained if we are to continue to serve others vigorously."

Now all this said, it was actually a story that this caring physician shared that really caught my attention:

"Truly embracing the concept of relationship-centered care, I try to honor this philosophy and approach in all of my encounters with patients.

One day I saw on my schedule that I would be meeting with Mrs. Smith (name changed). She is a 54-year-old, Caucasian woman who had seen members of my care team for 10 or so years but this was my first appointment with her.

I reviewed her file, her previous test results, her most recent test results, her MRIs over time, and I was so very excited to meet with her.

I walked in and introduced myself. I sat across from Mrs. Smith. We made and held eye contact, and we began to talk.

I learned more about Mrs. Smith, and she learned more about me. And after a good amount of sharing, I excitedly said,

'Mrs. Smith, I have reviewed all of your tests and I have great news. You do not have MS [multiple sclerosis].'

Well Tom, here I am thinking I am delivering wonderful news. But no.

Mrs. Smith was furious and was adamant that she had MS.

'Dr. Michaels said I have a touch of MS. He has been treating me for years. You must be wrong. I want to see MY doctor again!'

I couldn't believe it. I thought I had done the right thing. I researched her file. I ensured I introduced myself. I began to connect with Mrs. Smith. I was transparent. I assumed this would be good news. And that was one of my mistakes. I assumed.

As I said, this was my first time meeting Mrs. Smith. I had not established a relationship with her to date. I tried to connect during our (albeit limited) time together, but it was not enough. We did not have years of continuous learning and sharing together. I did not understand the emotional and mental aspects of her 'illness' and how they were being impacted. I did not realize her very identity was now so thoroughly connected to her illness (MS) that my news was actually devastating to her. I did not know.

Tom, this incident serves as a reminder to me that relationships cannot be hurried. Relationships take time. This situation also serves to remind me that the emotional, mental and spiritual dimensions of health and healing must be embraced by the care team. Only focusing on the physical aspect of health will inadvertently cause harm … like I did.

Looking back, if I could 'do-over' my visit with Mrs. Smith, I would have discussed her history with her in a far different way. We would have discussed the various dimensions of her health and healing. I would have sought deeper understanding. I would have leveraged my training, skills, intuition and wisdom and developed with Mrs. Smith a pathway that would have helped rather than harmed.

This is how I practice now. This is how I teach and this is how I lead. And as a healthcare leader it is my responsibility to build care models that promote this sort of approach to healing."

Needless to say, this sharing was passion fueled, from the heart, and a ripple for this chief experience officer to create a wave inside and outside of her healthcare institution.

It is also a reminder for me that we must evolve past patient-centered care and move toward relationship-centered care. We healthcare leaders must stop seeing our world with the blinders of what is and innovate to what should be.

> "There are those who look at things the way they are, and ask why … I dream of things that never were, and ask why not?" ~ RFK

And most importantly, it highlights that even with a great mission and intent, only when we are both humble and vulnerable and open to failing forward and learning will we truly be best positioned to both lead and serve and improve the lot of others.

Be courageous through your vulnerability and make a difference.

Questions

1. As a healthcare leader, when was the last time you "failed forward?" How did you embrace failing? What did you learn from the experience, and how did you apply these learnings to better serve others?

2. As a clinician or staff person, how often do you reflect on both your successes and your opportunities to do better? What tools do you use? How do you ensure you use this reflection time to learn and grow rather than beat yourself up? Please share a story of a time when you were successful in owning and learning from a mistake that you had made and, in doing so, also showed self-compassion.

3. As a patient or family member, when was the last time you heard "I am sorry" from a healthcare professional after he or she had made a mistake? What was that experience like? Please share a story.

4. How do we encourage courageous vulnerability in our efforts to lead and serve for the benefit of others? What would it look like?

Chapter 6

Back at It

The Fairfield Inn is basic but clean, quiet, and the staff courteous for all of us weary business travelers. The breakfast area was packed, but I was able to grab the last table and enjoy some melon and a steaming hot cup of coffee. Not Dunks mind you, but piping hot, nonetheless.

Okay. Now I am ready for work.

"Good morning, James. How was your evening?"

"Great. Patriots finally got a win last week after those three bad losses in a row. And for it to be against the Cowboys, all the better."

At this time, so early in our relationship, I figured I would not mention my affinity for the Cowboys. An authentic relationship is important … as is timing.

"Excellent. I am going to get settled and grab some more coffee. Then I would like to meet with the team in the small conference room at 9:00am."

"I will let them know."

And then, promptly at 9:00am, I knew I had my first opportunity to redeem my faux pas from the day before …

"Good morning, Team. I am so very thrilled to be back here with you all today. You each have already taught me a good deal and I look forward to much more learning and sharing with each of you."

After pausing to scan the room and looking into the eyes of each of my new teammates I continued, "One of the key reasons I wanted to be here, and there are a great many reasons, is to greatly improve access for our military members. For these folks to have to drive three hours for primary care services is unconscionable. From my review of this program, the access standards we are to honor include a maximum thirty-minute drive time for primary care and a sixty-minute drive time for specialty and ancillary services. Is this accurate?"

"Yes, Tom. That is our goal."

"The way I see it, this is a minimum standard. This is worst case. Our members should not have to drive sixty minutes to see a dermatologist or orthopedic surgeon or gynecologist. I wouldn't want that for my family, and we should not be satisfied with this for any of our members."

I continued ...

"So tell me, what have been the barriers to us honoring our commitment to these folks?"

"We have been pulled in many directions. There always seems to be a new strategy, a new process, a new initiative, a new ..." James hesitated for a moment prior to finishing his thought, "... flavor of the month. And each is resource intensive, and each takes us away from our mission to improve access."

"Thank you, James."

"Debbie?"

"I agree. Also, our fee schedule is really low."

"Yes. That is very true," James concurred.

"Please continue, Debbie. Tell me more about our fee schedule."

"We pay CMAC."

At first, I thought I was back in Brockton and someone was talking "smack."

"We pay what?"

I wanted to hear my team explain the current reimbursement system.

"We pay C – MAC," Debbie continued. "The Champus Maximum Allowable Charge. (CMAC)."

"Yes. I have read up on the Champus Rate. And I love acronyms. CMAC it is." I then added, "Why is CMAC a barrier? How does CMAC compare with Medicare and Medicaid rates in this market?"

"The CMAC rate is lower than both Medicare and Medicaid," Debbie responded.

"CMAC is lower than dirt," James added.

"I understand. So, the Department of Defense has set the rates for our program lower than dirt to manage unit costs. And you are saying that an unintended consequence of this level of payment to date here in Maine is the fact that we only have five primary care sites for all of our members living throughout the state of Maine and in Southern New Hampshire?"

"Exactly."

"And when we have built out the network of physicians, ancillaries, and hospitals for our members at a level where access is above the standards set by the feds, WHICH WE WILL, you are saying that due to these low payment levels, we will need to ensure we partner with our utilization management department to safeguard that our members are not over-treated (which can be just as harmful as under-treated) by practices who are trying to maximize their revenues by increasing the number of units … or in healthcare … by increasing the number of office visits and invasive procedures performed on our members?"

"Wait. No. We did not say that."

"And yet, that will be the case. Our commitment is to develop a network of high-quality and credentialed primary care and specialty care physicians and hospitals. We will be doing this using CMAC, as per the rules of engagement set by the DoD. We will be successful in doing this. AND, understanding how the healthcare system works and the desire for practices to maximize revenues, we will be cognizant of this fact and partner with our teammates in utilization management to ensure appropriate levels of care. Make sense?"

"Yes. Great sense. And I can work with them to analyze the utilization trends by physician, site, market, and specialty … anything we need."

"Fantastic, Jesse. That is exactly what we will need. And, in the meantime, we will need to develop by market a network access analytic tool so we can track our progress, share updates, and ensure we are honoring our commitments. We will want this for each specialty. When can you have a template for me?"

I remembered how much I love having an analyst in the department. And especially a dedicated, caring, mission-driven, brilliant one like Jesse.

"Mid next week?"

"Let's review an initial draft Tuesday afternoon."

"Denise, as you know, a provider directory is out of date as soon as it goes to print. We will be developing our expanded network efficiently and effectively over the next few months. Please think about what you will need to maintain the database as well as timing for updates. I want to ensure we are informing our members (and our teammates) in a timely fashion about updated access options. Let's get them care where they live and be sure they know it."

"Okay, Tom."

"Debbie, from our last discussion you mentioned your passion for provider relations and education. Please pull together all our current tools and your ideas to improve each for next week as well."

"Sounds good."

"James, what happens if one of our members sees a physician who is not contracted with us? What I mean is, what level of payment -- if any -- does the physician receive and is the patient responsible for any of it?"

"Hmmmm ... I believe that as long as the physician accepts Medicare, then they are not allowed to bill one of our members at all. And if, in fact, they do see one of our members, then the physician would be paid according to CMAC regardless."

"So you are saying whether they contract with us or not, they are being paid the same for seeing one of our military members?"

"Yes. That is right."

"And you said CMAC is less than dirt."

"Right again."

"So, clearly (and unlike many other managed care companies), we are not going to be able to contract with them based on price?"

"That is the issue."

I loved seeing Debbie already coming out of her shell.

"And again whether they contract with us or not, they get paid the same for seeing our members. So here is the deal ... It is my job to eliminate barriers that prevent you all from doing your job. I will ensure no "flavor of the month" and no "bright shiny new object" pulls you away from honoring our commitment to our members. And together, we will no longer try to contract with physicians and hospitals based on price."

"The first part sounds good. But the second ..."

It is never a bad thing to have a caring and passionate skeptic in the room. In fact, I loved it. They test, they push, and they ensure nothing is overlooked.

"Hear me out, James. Banging your head against the wall over and over again will only give you a headache. You all have worked incredibly hard to build networks of physicians, while being pulled in numerous misaligned directions and negotiating a non-negotiable low reimbursement. Moving forward, we do not lose focus, and we take the low reimbursement issue off the table. In fact, what we do is we offer upfront that our reimbursement is extremely low, it is mandated, that they receive it whether they contract or not, and that there is no negotiating this point."

"We steal their negotiating thunder."

"Exactly, Jesse. We then focus on what brought many of us here … which is honoring our commitments to those who have served in the military. We focus on why it is important to do so. We focus on the lack of access. We focus on patient safety. We focus on quality of care. We focus on mission and heart and compassion. We focus on the 'why.'"

I recall at this point thinking about the lesson I learned the day prior and carefully balancing my passion with the fact that I was not military and many of those I was partnering with were.

"But what if they say no?"

"We won't worry about that at this time, Denise. As a team, we are going to honor our commitments. As a team, we will focus on supporting military dependents and military retirees. As a team, we will stop negotiating price. And as a team, we will surpass our goals by focusing on the why. I believe people are honorable … even if occasionally they need to be reminded of what truly matters."

"Agreed?"

"YES!"

"Excellent. Now I will be meeting with the utilization management and the credentialing team today. I want to ensure we are all on the same page in this effort. That all departments, all teams, are aware of our aim, our focus, our approach, and quite frankly how very busy we are all going to be quite soon."

After the team headed back to their cubicles, I remained in the conference room and processed our discussion.

I loved the energy in the room. And I loved how each team member seemed to simply want a clear mission and someone who believed in it … and in them. These are good people and it appears (so far) that the system has been designed to achieve the current poor results (as they say in quality improvement speak) rather than these people not being able to do the job. In fact, so far, I believe these people are perfect for the job, and it is my job to engage and lead them … and to fix the system. So far so good.

And with that I headed out of the conference room.

"Hey James." He and I met unexpectedly in the men's room. "Are you clear on your next steps?"

"Oh yes. Got it." And then a pause. "I really appreciate your candor, insight, and passion. It has been missing around here for a long time."

Gratitude too? I think I am going to love this team, I remember saying to myself before cautiously responding, "I truly believe in what we need to accomplish. That is why I am here."

"I know, Tom. I know."

REFLECTION

Back in the early 1990s, while working for a well-respected managed care plan, I was involved in the implementation of quality-based incentive programs (now called pay-for-performance or P4P programs) where we incentivized physicians and medical practices to do certain things such as improve patient satisfaction and adhere to a drug formulary.

Some years later, I developed these incentive models and oversaw their use and impact. And over time, I learned a great deal about controllable outcomes, unintended consequences, and the direct and indirect impacts of such models.

Now 20+ years later, as we continue to move from productivity-based reimbursement to quality-based reimbursement via the accountable care organization and other payment reform models, a large caution sign is illuminated before me.

Recently, I was speaking with a former colleague who had decided to leave the nonprofit sector within the healthcare system to go back to school. She is now at Boston University in what sounds like a very interesting MBA program and is apparently learning a great deal more of the business side of nonprofits.

> *"Yes, Tom, we are studying the impact of incentivizing behaviors, and I must admit that during our most recent project there was definitely an adrenaline rush having to do with both chasing and receiving a financial reward for achieving a specific target."*

> *"But do you really want a physician to be driven to care because they are chasing a financial reward as opposed to the fact that they actually truly care?"*

> *"But, Tom, what if a financial incentive does actually bring about positive change?"*

And of course. this led me to the Harvard Business Review and the piece "Why Incentive Plans Cannot Work":

> *1. Rewards do not create a lasting commitment. They merely, and temporarily, change what we do.*

> *2. People are likely to become less interested in their work, requiring extrinsic incentives before expending effort.*

In addition, it's very important to me as a patient, as a family member, and as a healthcare leader to know that those who are caring for those I love are doing so because they truly care – and not because they are being financially incentivized to do so. And as a parent who has lived the fear of a child living her first few days in the NICU, I know that I would want (did want/do want) the person caring for my baby to be someone who does just that – truly and authentically care – rather than someone who is motivated by an additional financial return for pretending to do so.

Yes, perhaps the financial incentives will change behavior (temporarily), and perhaps they will even have an impact on HCAHPS and other satisfaction and experience scores. But even if those scores were not affected only temporarily, do we really want a healthcare system to be driven by financial rewards rather than an enduring commitment to quality and safety by people who truly care?

Financial incentives may temporarily change outcomes, but they do not change hearts.

- *We must not edge the humanity out of healthcare via over reliance on financial drivers of change.*

- *We must focus on changing adaptively rather than with a quick financially based technical fix.*

- *We must focus on bringing humanity back into healthcare once again.*

- *We must eliminate existing barriers to true caring.*

And as we do so, let's ensure that we position doctors, nurses, and all participants within the healthcare system to authentically care about one another and themselves so that we all feel cared for and cared about. For when we are all whole and healthy, we will be best positioned to care for one another.

True healthCARING will be long lasting and will truly innovate healthcare.

Like the old saying goes, "money can't buy love."

Or in this case, "financial drivers can't buy sustainable or authentic caring."

Questions

1. As a healthcare leader, clinician, or staff person, how often have you found yourself or your team losing focus on your mission, your goal, and your aim due to the "shiny new nickel" syndrome?
2. As a healthcare leader, what have you done to ensure distractions do not pull you away from your personal and professional mission?
3. As a healthcare leader, how often do you embrace the skeptic in the room?
4. As a healthcare leader, clinician, or staff person, how do you ensure you remain open to new ideas? To being wrong?
5. As a healthcare leader, clinician, or staff person, what unintended consequences of various payment methodologies have you witnessed?
    a. What would you do to address them?
    b. Which payment model(s) would you recommend and why?
6. Should there be financial incentive to do the right thing? What is the upside? What is the downside?
    a. Can people truly and authentically be financially incentivized to care? Should they be?

Chapter 7

Progress

The weekend home was not as relaxing as I had hoped.

Nope. We had moving to do. Or at least the continued preparation for the big day when we move our pentad plus Angus north to Alaska. (Doc continued to believe Maine was Alaska even after our multiple visits there together.)

"We might as well be moving to Alaska!" was frequently spoken as we carted rubbish to the dump, made piles for Goodwill, and wrapped treasures in bubble wrap.

"Do you want these trophies? I found them in the attic."

My baseball trophies. Two league championships and a city-wide championship. One to which I contributed greatly. The others were the year I was progressed way too fast. Skipping over an entire league (where my brother was excelling prior to hurting his elbow) to move into the majors and play with kids much older than me. Did the move feed my ego? You bet. Did it feel good to surpass my brother the better athlete? Oh yes. Was it a bad move? Hard to answer. I learned a lot from the experience, which I have used to coach my son and other young men in sports as well as my work teams. But was it exceedingly hard on me as a young man? Definitely. I believe I set the record (at least in my own mind) for errors in my first season in the majors, and my hitting was just as poor. But again, looking back years later as an adult, I learned so much that I use to this day to help others I cannot say it was a bad move.

"No dear. You can toss them."

Looking back now, perhaps I should have kept them as a reminder of the team's accomplishments and even more so of the trials and the lessons learned from those challenging times.

By Monday morning I was ready to head back to Maine (again without my family) and to face the challenges side by side with my new team.

Doc and I had just said our goodbyes after she had gotten up early to make me coffee and breakfast.

"Being away from you for a week this time is going to be so hard."

"For me too, but I will be busy with the kids and getting the rest of our packing done. And you will be busy saving the world."

The ride north that morning gave me that "in my head" time I needed to process much of what was happening and what needed to be done. And the Dunks coffee with cream and no sugar helped a great deal, too.

As I approached Randolph, traffic began to pick up, and my recent acceleration dampened. But not my processing.

Our mission, and my vision, are all important. But in this case, and with the organization having such a poor track record of honoring the military families specific to access outside of the core markets, this needs to be about action. Action to eliminate barriers and action to achieve the mission. Period.

I also recall continuing to try to leverage the learning from my mistakes from the week prior.

I need to be mindful that we are all coming at this from different places, we are all very different people, and we are all bringing our own shadow (the good stuff and the not so good stuff). Each interaction (whether perceived immediately as good or bad) is an opportunity to garner new information and learn from it. It is not personal. My focus must stay on the True North. On the mission. And my heart must focus on being open to new ideas and new wisdom.

I was getting pumped, similar to the feeling just prior to leaving the locker room in college. And lucky for me the traffic had lightened a bit as Route 24 North joined Route 128 South, and I began to accelerate again.

"Stay on target!" I joked as I quoted Star Wars and turned onto interstate 93 North.

And two and a half hours later I was pulling back into the parking lot at my office.

"Good morning, Debbie. Did you have a nice weekend?"

"Good morning, Tom. Yes. Lots of time with my two pups."

Debbie and I spoke a bit, and I learned a great deal more about her through her stories of her animals and also her inquiries into my animals and family. She truly is someone who cares deeply. Someone who wants to learn. Someone who I was blessed to have on my team.

"We have much to do. Are you ready?"

And with a big wonderful smile, "Oh yes, Tom. Very!"

And over the next six months, using the strategy we developed together, and leveraging the heart and passions of our team, we developed a network of contracted providers meeting or exceeding the DoD access standards in each of our markets. Yes, in six months with focus (eliminating all barriers) and teamwork, these amazing people achieved more than had been done in the prior fifteen years.

Together, we honored our mission to the military families. And together, we also became a family.

I also got to know Esther far beyond our initial sharing and disconnect. And I confirmed that she truly is an amazing and caring person who I trust and respect as a professional and enjoy as a friend.

I got to see James beyond the organization. Yes, he is a high-character, high-integrity professional who cares deeply about his team and mission. And he is an amazing dad and husband who loves his family beyond description. A hard charger with great intensity and strength.

Jesse, too. Not only a dedicated, passionate, mission-driven professional, but also another high-integrity, high-character family man. Brilliant. Calming. A true team player.

Debbie continued to shine. To bring her heart and mind and soul into all she did. To pick up her teammates and teach as much as she learned. Driven. Heart-centered. Servant leader.

And Denise, holding the team together with her in-house administrative focus, wry sense of humor, and energy.

And of course, our team branched beyond the five of us and Esther. We engaged Marie and her medical management team, Claire and Stephen in marketing / member services, Beth in credentialing, and so many other high caliber teammates all seeking to improve the organization and better position all of our members (new and old) for better health.

Truly a remarkable team. And truly a remarkable accomplishment.

"Congratulations, Tom, on a tremendous feat."

"Thank you, Saul. The team is amazing. They simply needed a direction and some barriers removed and they did it."

Saul, the CEO and President of the organization, responded with some niceties directed at me, but like many, I was challenged to hear and accept them.

"So Tom, the practices need some help."

Oh well, so much for the compliments, I remember thinking.

"As you know we are both a payer, with our military program, and a provider, via our four owned practice locations. The contracts our sites have with the managed care plans are not financially beneficial to the organization, they are also unwieldy, and at the end of the day no one is really managing them."

In fact, I learned, the contracts were sitting in a box under one employee's desk.

> TIP: If you ever are looking for lost contracts, be sure to look under everyone's desk.

"Now that you have the network built for our military families…"

"Saul, there is still plenty more to do."

"I know, I know, but you and your team will get it done. So, as I was saying, now that you have the network built, I would like you to take on the responsibility for negotiating and managing all of the practices' managed care contracts. You know, in your spare time."

I thought Saul was joking about my 'spare time.' But perhaps not.

"You have the background for it. You have a great team now in place for the military work. This will be a promotion of course."

I remember getting the impression that this was more of a demand than a request. Or as they said in the Godfather, "an offer I could not refuse." That said, I actually thought this would be a great deal of fun. I would be able to represent the organization as part of the local Physician Hospital Organization (PHO) payer negotiating committee, work for both the military healthcare program and the practices, see two sides of the healthcare equation (payer and provider) at the same time, and expand my knowledge while also being of service and providing more value in a whole new way.

[NOTE: In my opinion, PHOs should be referred to as HPOs (HiPPOs) based on where the real decision authority lives, but that is for another discussion.]

"Saul, I would love this new responsibility. Count me in."

But of course, as soon as I said it, I knew I could be in a bit a trouble at home. Doc understands my passions, but she was always concerned about me taking on too much.

"Wonderful, Tom. You can find the contracts in a box ..."

I almost laughed out loud.

During these six months, Doc and I moved our family from Massachusetts to Maine. We spent our first Christmas away from family and began new traditions with my cousins and other extended family nearby. The kids began school, and we learned that a Maine winter (southern Maine anyway) was not that much different than a Massachusetts winter. At least in the year 2000. Alaska, Maine was not.

And then later that summer ...

"Tom, you haven't taken on too much have you?"

"No. The team is amazing. I am so enjoying working with Sandy in the practices and collaborating with Paul from the PHO. I now understand far better the folks I work with and their passions. And each day I am reinvigorated."

"But you look so tired."

"Nah. I am so excited to go to work each day."

"And what about what happened at the gym?"

"What do you mean?"

"Don't play dumb. You know what happened."

"It was nothing. I was just tired."

"No ..."

Doc had that look on her face.

"... chest pains and needing to lay down across the two front seats in your car after a workout is not 'NOTHING'!"

"Honey ..."

"Don't you 'honey' me!"

"Doc, I was just tired. It was 'Leg Day.'"

I almost laughed with all the jokes over the years we made about 'Chest Day' and 'Leg Day'.

"I had done a ton of squats."

"You did squats with those knees!"

I was clearly not helping my own cause.

"Okay. Okay. I still say it was nothing … but I will take it easy this weekend. No gym. Let's just go do something fun with the kids. How about the beach?"

"The beach in Maine in June?! This is Alaska!"

Apparently, there was no way I was going to win the argument. The only hope was to get out of it alive.

"What would you like to do?"

"You just take it easy. I love you. What happened at the gym is not 'nothing.' And you are not leaving me alone with the kids here in Maine. Understood?"

REFLECTION

A team full of heart and passion can overcome a lousy or non-existent strategic plan.

A solid strategic plan will never overcome a team lacking heart and passion.

Questions

1. As a healthcare leader, clinician, staff person, patient, or family member, reflecting back on your childhood were there challenges that you faced either successfully or unsuccessfully that you tap into as an adult?
    a. What lessons were learned?
    b. How have you applied those lessons as an adult to benefit others?
2. As a clinician, staff person, patient, or family member, is it a challenge for you to truly accept a compliment?
    a. Do you take the time to hold the feedback in your heart as you cherish yourself? Why or why not?
    b. What would you recommend to those you lead relative to the importance of accepting an authentic compliment?
3. As a healthcare leader, clinician, or staff person, do you believe a high functioning team can also be like a family or do you believe that crosses a line? Why?
4. How about love? Is love important in healthcare? In business? Is love key to being a successful leader?
5. How have you improved the "teamness" within your organization?
    a. What would you recommend to other leaders relative to improving "teamness"?

Chapter 8

Taking on too much

"You will make a fine Chief Operating Officer."

I remember thinking, *Me, the COO of our military healthcare program?*

I had been at this organization for just over one and a half years. Yes, my team had done amazing work to honor our mission to military families. The network had been greatly expanded with credentialed physicians and hospitals. We were now focusing on further improving our access to services such as dermatology. (Which, quite frankly, was such a surprise to me that access specifically to dermatology was such an issue throughout Maine. In Massachusetts that was typically not the case, but lesson re-learned, each market is different). My team had continued to amaze, and our relationship with our peers in medical management, quality, claims, membership services, marketing and other key areas had grown strong.

On the payer front, the practices were better positioned with many newly negotiated managed care contracts either through the Maine Medical Center PHO contracting committee (which I loved serving on) or through direct negotiations.

Yes, I was tired but also feeling very blessed to be part of such a special community here. And now Rebus, our CFO, was telling me he thought I would be a fine COO for the plan.

"Thank you, Rebus. What is Saul's thinking?"

"Saul wants to reorganize his direct reports so that he can focus more on his vision. And that would mean he will need more capacity to focus on connecting directly with politicos, other leaders across the country and perhaps beyond … more of an outward focus."

His intention made great sense to me.

"That would mean he would have less time for direct interaction with the practices and the military program. His thought is to bring in a Practice Chief and a Plan Chief. That way, all functions within the practices and within the plan would report to each of these COOs. They would be responsible for all aspects of the respective business lines including Profit and Loss, Quality, Growth, etc."

Now this was getting interesting I remember thinking. And as Rebus continued, I remember my juices flowing with a new excitement. Plus of course the ever present, 'what will Doc say?' in the back of my mind.

"Would this role be of interest to you, Tom?"

With my introverted preference, I process much internally and typically only after having looked at a situation from a number of different perspectives would be ready to share verbally. But in this case, I kept hearing in my head 'lost opportunity' … and as I said, 'what will Doc say?' (Doc was truly my thought partner and had a keen intellect married with a great intuition.)

At this time, she already believed I had taken on too much. But this was an opportunity for me to continue to serve this population and my team (expanded team with the full plan staff) and to have a greater impact. To be of service in a different and greater way for our military families.

"Rebus, this role would be amazing. The restructuring makes great sense. And I believe my skills and passions align very well."

"I do too, Tom. Saul is planning a national recruitment effort but as I said, I believe you would be a fine candidate."

Now how was I going to tell Doc?

Later that evening …

"Doc, now that the kids are in bed …"

"Uh oh."

"Seriously. I want to talk to you about something that happened at work today."

"That is why I am 'uh oh-ing'. What did you take on now?"

Sometimes it was scary how well she knew me.

"Saul is restructuring. He wants to focus more on driving his vision and being externally focused."

"What did you do?" came Doc's response with not even a hint of a smile.

Damn.

"Honey."

"Don't 'honey' me. What did you do?"

"Listen, Saul's external focus will mean there may be an opportunity for me to take on a larger role and have a greater impact than what I am currently doing."

"And?"

Doc was clearly not making this easy.

"It looks like there will be a Chief Operating Officer position created for both the practices and for the military program."

"And you want this role?"

"I spoke with Rebus today. He shared some confidence in me in this role."

"But he doesn't have to take care of you when you break down because you took on too much. You do it all the time. And who is there to take care of you when you are up all night in pain? When your head is about to explode? When you cannot lay on your shoulder? When your stress level is over the top? Not Rebus."

She is right, of course. I have learned over the years that she is usually (okay, always) right.

"I know. I know. But this is different, my love."

"Don't you, 'my love,' me! And this is not different. This is the same. You do it all the time. Just like at Beech Street when you came home to tell me that you were going to be running offices in both Massachusetts AND New Jersey and that you were going to be developing workers' compensation networks well beyond the original New England territory you were initially responsible for. How was your health then? Who rubbed your shoulder and helped you get through those nightly migraines when you couldn't sleep? Not Rebus!"

I realized I had clearly learned very little when sharing these things with Doc.

"Honey." And before she could say it, "Yes, I am 'honeying' you. I really believe this is right for me. It is an opportunity to lead the entire military program. It is an opportunity to position even more amazing people to do the amazing things they are capable of … just like my network development team. I believe this is right for me. And besides, it may not even happen. Saul is doing a search and I may not even get the role."

Yes, I had tears in my eyes as I expressed from my heart my desire to move in this direction and ideally do more good.

"Rebus apparently is putting in a good word for me, but my guess is the odds are against it as Saul tends to like to bring in new blood."

"Who are you kidding? You know you will get it if you want it."

Now that is why I love her.

"I just want you with me. I need you to be okay with this if, in fact, Saul promotes me to this role."

"We both know you are going to do it regardless. You never listen to me."

At least she was smiling now.

The next day I must admit this new role was greatly on my mind.

"Tom."

"Yes, Saul."

For the next couple of hours Saul and I discussed the re-engineering and his intention to spread throughout the organization the quality management principles we had learned at the Center for Quality Management (CQM) in Cambridge.

> [CQM was founded in 1989 by seven companies in the Boston area in order to facilitate mutual learning of Total Quality Management and accelerate its implementation. Some of these seven companies included Bose Corporation, GE Aircraft Engine, Teradyne Incorporated, and Polaroid.]

Saul's idea had been to bring quality improvement principles from industry to healthcare. And he set out to do it by having many of us trained in TQM.

Over the previous year or so I, along with a number of other leaders throughout the organization, learned Root Cause Analysis (RCA), PDSA, the 7-Step Problem Solving Method, Mobilizing Change Using the 7 Infrastructures, the Method for Priority Marking, Language Processing, Leading without Authority, Concept Engineering, and the Voice of the Customer, and so much more.

The training (which also created great opportunity for team building) was brilliant as were the learnings and the impact of these learnings in practice.

In fact, at one point we saved much staffing expense when a team I was leading leveraged the learned QI tools and processes to increase efficiency and customer satisfaction relative to claims inquiries from one of our key hospitals.

We then discussed his overall vision. His goals for the re-engineering. His expectations and his intentions and then, with very little segue, he asked me to share with him my interest level in the COO role.

Quite frankly, I had all I could do to not jump up and say, "This is the role of my dreams! I will position our team to do great things. We will greatly and positively impact all those we serve, and you will be so very pleased."

But with Doc's voice in my head, I simply let Saul know that I believe the re-engineering made great sense, I appreciate and respect his vision and his willingness to share it with me, and that I have great interest in the role and believe I would provide value.

"Good to know, Tom. I appreciate you listening and your interest."

Honestly, I would have preferred more enthusiasm than that, but perhaps we were both keeping our cards close to the vest?

And then later that evening …

"Doc, I spoke to Saul."

"Yeah?"

Again, not the enthusiasm I was hoping for. But then again, I should not have expected it in either case.

"I can see Saul's vision. It makes great sense. And I know I am fairly young …"

> *As I spoke, I remembered a few years prior when I worked at a law firm a peer telling me at that time, "You are 32 years old. You are a kid to most of the attorneys, doctors and healthcare leaders you will be working with. You need to prove they should listen to you."*

"… but I believe I can make a difference. I want to try, honey. I want this role."

"Tom, listen to me. I know you do. And if it is meant to be, you will get it. Either now or in a few years when you are older."

As always, my bride ended up being supportive and saying exactly what I needed to hear.

"Now go get the kids. It is time for dinner."

"Sammy, Tommy, Haylee! I am coming to get you!" I shouted with a chuckle as I ran up the stairs.

"Daddy!!!!!"

About a week later Saul called me into his office …

"Tom. I have been doing a lot of thinking."

Darn it. Not a good sign.

"I believe you will be a fine COO for our military program."

Oh my god. He is offering me the promotion.

"I have spoken with Lisa, we have put together a job description and salary range for this role. And, I am officially offering it to you."

"Breathe, Tom. Breathe," I reminded myself.

We then discussed Saul's expectations and goals for the person in this role. And after fleshing it out a bit further I responded, "Thank you, Saul. This is so exciting. I will review everything with my bride and give you my final decision tomorrow. This is life changing."

Little did I know.

REFLECTION

I have had the privilege of coaching amazing young men in a high school recreation basketball league for a good many years.

And I remember one particular game where we were getting beat soundly, and our players were feeling pretty down. I remember turning and looking up at the scoreboard and seeing we were trailing 43 to 12 late in the first half, and I remember calling our players' attention to it.

I called their attention to the fact that the outside world was judging us based on those electric red numbers glaring ... and yet the outside world had no idea the measure of a young man's heart, the real measure of our team's success.

We turned our attention toward each of our own measures of success, each step we were making individually and together to improve as basketball players (and coaches) and as men. We talked about the outside world and the glare of the red, and set that aside to focus on the REAL wins, the TRUE measures of success.

Back on the court, the other team continued driving, scoring, pushing, harassing, showboating and taunting. And yet my boys never gave an inch and played with perseverance, tenacity, and integrity until the final whistle.

And even though the neon red numbers had grown further and further apart, by the end of the game they no longer glared down on our team. Those numbers were no longer the key metric to be measured against; they were no longer all encompassing.

In fact, the outside world's view changed for that one game, and it saw what the glowing red numbers could never show, as exemplified by the two referees approaching me after the game and saying, "Those boys ... we have never seen that type of maturity, focus, determination and HEART in all of our years of refereeing than we saw tonight. What an amazing team. What fine young men."

When I am challenged at work, I often look back on that one incredible game and think about what those young men taught me and how I can use those lessons in the midst of a healthcare world that judges based on metrics that may not be the true measure of success.

In fact, not too long ago I again mulled this all over as I was developing measures of success for a partner organization. I had seen this organization evolve and grow under great leadership. I had also seen their measures of success that are truly amazing, and yet clearly not what the outside world wanted to see. And again, I reflected back on that special night.

As you look at your own organization, your team, your family, yourself, as you review your organization's vision and mission, your team's and your family's goals, and perhaps your own vision and mission, how are you measuring success?

Measuring success is critical to achieving success. — "You cannot manage what you cannot measure." — Defining success is just as critical. The next time you look into the eyes of your board, your funder(s), your staff, your patients, your customers, your team, your family ... the next time you as a leader look in the mirror, be sure you have a clear definition of success (and a way to measure it) to ensure you know the pathway to achieving the defined success.

The delivery of optimal healthcare will continue to be full of challenges and yet these challenges can and will be mitigated by leaders who mindfully define, measure and manage their own success and the success of their team and organization ... with Heart.

One final note: Beware of those red numbers glaring in your eyes. They may not be what really matters.

Questions

1. As a healthcare leader, clinician, or staff person, have you leveraged tools from other industries, such as TQM, Lean, Six Sigma, and others to improve healthcare in your institution?
    a. What were the major barriers in doing so?
    b. What were the benefits?
    c. What lessons learned and best practices did you garner?
    d. Did leadership buy in? How did you engage them?
    e. What would you suggest to someone in another healthcare organization who has interest in moving in this direction?
    f. What would be the first thing you would recommend they do?
2. As a healthcare leader, clinician, staff person, patient, or family member, do you have a thought partner in your life?
    a. Who do you share your greatest triumphs with? Your recent failures? Your fears?
    b. Do you believe it is important to have someone you can talk to about anything? Why? Why not?
    c. What would you suggest to someone if they do not have a thought partner?

Chapter 9

Voice of the Customer

"Tom, we need to add a dental benefit for our military members and patients."

Even though I had been here for well over a year, as the new COO for the military healthcare program, I was still getting used to having former peers as either direct reports or as direct reports to my counterpart on the Practice side, Sandy Fortis, the Practice COO. That said, my relationship with Claire Captiosus, Director of Marketing, was no different than it had been.

Claire is brilliant and a fast thinker and talker. She has strong instincts, is business savvy, and is also a great deal of fun to work with.

"What makes you think we need to add a dental benefit? How do you know, Claire? And what is the goal?"

"The goal is to increase membership. I know we need a dental benefit because that is what the focus groups told us."

I have a bias when it comes to focus groups. They can easily be manipulated to give you the result you want and thus the details and the process must be analyzed closely.

"Tell me more about the focus groups."

Claire went into fine detail as to the mechanics including sharing, "So when existing and potential members have a choice of new benefits such as an eye care benefit or dental benefit, they overwhelmingly choose a dental benefit."

"Claire, I have read the focus group reports. And some of the key points that stuck out for me included quotes such as, 'I want to see a doctor who listens to me' and 'I can get seen when I need to be seen, in a timely matter.'"

I continued …

"I also read in the June 2000 focus group report, which you also did a great job developing, that our existing patients believe quality healthcare means such things as …

1. Communicating with and listening to patients
2. Being thorough
3. Having patients participate in their care
4. Being an advocate for the patient's care
5. Developing good relationships between patient and provider
6. Seeing the same doctor consistently
7. Being seen as a whole person, not as a collection of parts
8. Being treated respectfully
9. Having coordinated care
10. And much more

… but nowhere did I read anything about a dental benefit."

"Tom, in the data, in the details of the data, it is clear that when benefits are discussed, the dental benefit is the highest priority for existing and potential new members."

We had just invested a great deal of time, money, and energy in quality improvement training. And part of the training included learning the Voice of the Customer qualitative data analysis approach (or VoC) to engage those whose interest we in the military healthcare program represent and whose perspective can add value to our understanding and decision-making.

"I understand we have focus group data, Claire. And we need to turn this data into information and the information into wisdom, not only for you and me, but for people throughout the organization, including Saul. What I am suggesting is we implement a VoC process to confirm (or not) the findings of the focus groups you conducted. And in doing so, we will also be getting value out of our CQM investment (which will please Saul and Rebus) and will further engage them in this process."

And after much discussion between two individuals who truly respect and trust one another I asked, "Does that make sense to you?"

"Actually Tom, that does make sense. Especially the part of getting Saul's and Rebus's attention."

"Excellent. I am meeting with Saul in the morning. I will share with him our discussion and our collective intention to move forward with the VoC, and ideally he will buy in."

Later as I re-read the focus group data, I was even more impressed with it and also very aware that there had been little movement in truly addressing many of the quality of care and other important items identified. And with the new pressures throughout the healthcare system to move to even shorter office visits in order to maximize revenues, I believed more so of the need to ensure we were truly hearing the voices of our patients and members as we sought to improve the healthcare delivery model. Ideally, I thought, this VoC process will assist us in this effort.

My gut also told me that adding a dental benefit and service (while very easy in the grand scheme of things) was not going to significantly improve care quality, nor would it truly meet our needs relative to member acquisition and growth (which was the major driver of moving in this direction).

"We can do better. We must do better. It is our mission to do better," I thought. And as COO for the military program, I felt it was my responsibility to make sure of it and thus nail the meeting with Saul in the morning.

"What is that smell?"

It was 4:30am the next morning.

"I am not sure, Doc. It is not me."

"Ha ha ha, I know. Is the window open?"

"Yes. And it smells like a skunk to me. Either a skunk or great coffee."

"You do like your coffee strong don't you?"

"You know it. And I am going to need it this morning."

"Why?"

I had been up all-night thinking about the meeting with Saul this morning. I was continuing to try to counterbalance the predominantly financial pressures from throughout the healthcare system to maximize revenues at the expense of patient safety and quality of care. And so far, the straightforward approach and other strategies I had tried to implement had not worked. My goal on this morning was to leverage Saul's strong desire for the organization to utilize and leverage quality improvement principles to improve how we provide service and care to our members and our patients. I believed if I could convince Saul to greenlight me leading a team to truly listen and honor the voices of our members and patients via the Voice of the Customer process, the outcomes would show that the financial drivers pushing healthcare institutions toward more and more technology and shorter and shorter office visits would be offset by the loss of members and patients and worse care quality, safety, and outcomes.

I did not want our organization to follow the path of so many others.

So, this early morning, with the smell of skunk seeping through the open window, I explained this to Doc.

"Tom, it is way too early to be following all of that. All I know is you have a good heart, and you are wicked smart." I always love when Doc's Brockton comes out. "And you need to sleep at night, or you are going to get sick."

"Good morning, Saul."

"Good morning, Tom. How was your night?"

I remember thinking, "Hmmmm … I don't think I will mention the skunk or the lack of sleep (although the puffiness and dark circles under my eyes will probably be a tell)."

"It was a very nice night, Saul. Doc made a big spaghetti dinner and I got to bathe Haylee in the kitchen sink afterwards. I believe she wore more homemade sauce then she ate."

"Ha ha ha. Nothing like family time."

"How about you?"

"Well, less family time than I would prefer. I met with a very interesting physician from up north over dinner."

Saul was always meeting very interesting and typically brilliant people in an effort to acquire new information to not only improve his own understanding of a specific topic or to learn something new but also to improve the organization. Which I admired greatly. He was truly a knowledge-seeker for the right reasons.

"Saul, there are many reasons to grow the our military healthcare organization with the utmost in my mind being to provide additional access to high-quality and credentialed physicians for those we serve."

"Absolutely. So, what are you driving at?"

"I have been reviewing the recent focus group data with Claire. Claire believes that a key strategy to increasing our census is to add a new benefit. A dental benefit to be exact."

"Yes. She has shared these same data with me as well."

Hmmmm ... not sure if that is a good thing or not.

"Saul, I believe through our partnership with the Center for Quality Management we now have an opportunity to leverage our learnings and the tools they have shared to truly assess the key drivers (and barriers) of growth for us. And if, in fact, it is a new dental benefit, so be it. But perhaps it is something else."

"So what are you proposing?"

Right to the point. This is good.

"Saul, I am proposing that I pull together a cross-functional team, and we conduct a Voice of the Customer project. We gather and truly hear the voices of members and patients who love us, those who hate us, and more. We follow the process. We listen to the stories from these people and through the Language Processing method, we identify and prioritize key requirements for future growth."

"How long will this take?"

"Give me 30 days, and I will provide you with a prioritized list of requirements using this market-in approach."

"What about the focus groups? What about that expense? What about those data?"

As Claire and I had discussed, I shared with Saul the fact that in a typical VoC process the data collected is verified through a mindfully developed and administered survey tool or focus group. I said that in our case, we simply reverse the order. We had the focus group data already. Now we conduct the VoC. We verify and get it right. We move forward into action. This way our existing investment would not be lost and, in fact, is part of our evolved process. I also highlighted the fact that we would be leveraging our investment in CQM. And at the end of the day, we would have better data.

"Hmmmm ... you have certainly thought this through."

"Saul, it is very important to me that we continue to provide those we serve with access to better care."

"What about Claire? She is invested in moving forward with a dental benefit. And I am thinking that when we do ..."

When we do? Darn it. I was clearly not swaying Saul, I thought.

"... we will also add a dental service in our clinic to ensure high quality care and keep the funding stream in-house."

I took a deep breath and ensured I kept my voice steady even as my passion for doing this right was beginning to take over.

"Saul …"

Breathe Tom. Breathe, I reminded myself.

"… Claire and I discussed this evolved approach in detail yesterday. And I hear where she is coming from. And she hears where I am coming from. She agrees with this new approach. And she believes a thirty-day window would actually work quite well."

I took another breath.

"Saul, I understand analysis paralysis. I don't see this fitting that definition. We have a plan. I have my team identified. Claire is bought in. We will actually be generating more value from our investment in both the focus groups and the CQM training. And we will get this right by listening and honoring the voices of those we serve."

I continued …

"We will also be showing the organization that we leaders are walking our talk, that we are engaging in a quality improvement effort, and we are using what we learned from CQM. We will be generating a return on investment all while doing what is right."

"Tom …"

Saul and I discussed my proposal for the rest of our meeting. He, as always, was very thorough in his analysis and asked great questions.

Personally, I felt like I was on a bit of a roller coaster. Some questions led me to believe he wanted to proceed directly to a new benefit. Other questions felt like we were going to proceed with the Voice of the Customer project.

And after another twenty minutes or so …

"Tom, make it happen. Pull together your team and conduct the Voice of the Customer. Let's hear our patients' and members' voices. Their stories. From these stories, develop a prioritized list of requirements. Then verify the requirements with the previously completed focus groups and have a final report to me in thirty days."

Thirty days? I said to myself. *What was I thinking?*

"Yes, sir. I will have the team in place by the end of the day and will expedite making this happen. And if, in fact, the data comes back and points to adding a dental benefit … then that is what we will do."

And on the way back to my office from Portland …

"Hey Doc."

"I thought you were meeting with Saul this morning."

"We just finished. I am driving back to my office."

"How did it go?"

"Well, I got what I wanted."

"Ha ha ha … don't you always?"

God, I love her and her Dahlborg sense of humor.

"You know that old saying, 'be careful what you wish for, you just might get it'?"

"Yes."

"Well, I have thirty days to lead a cross-functional team to conduct a Voice of the Customer project, which is a process none of us has ever done. With everyone already at or very near full capacity or beyond."

"Then why did you push for this?"

Like Saul she is right to the point.

"Because I don't believe that adding a dental benefit will significantly impact our ability to improve access to our program. And if we are not successful, fewer military families will know of and engage with a healthcare program I believe is better than any out there."

"So as usual you took on more than you should have."

I remember arriving back at my office and seeing James at the coffee machine.

"James, we have improved access by expanding the network successfully. And now we are going to determine how best to engage with our existing and future members and patients and create pathways for them to access our expanded network and program."

"What is your timeline?"

"Thirty days."

"That is tight."

"And I am going to need you and the rest of our team to continue to do your amazing work while I am focusing in this space."

"You know we have your back."

Yes, I did. Always. Be it James's military background or the fact that I was blessed with an amazing team (probably both), I knew they had each other's backs, they had my back, and I hope they knew I had theirs.

And as I walked away from James I thought about the fact that not only were we supporting one another, but we were doing so because we truly believed in our mission, to support and help all those we serve. We cared about each other, and we were crystal clear as to our higher purpose.

"Claire!" I called ahead as I saw her heading down the hallway toward the medical management department.

"Saul greenlighted our VoC."

"That is great!"

Claire was all set to proceed with adding a dental benefit based on all the data she had collected and analyzed to date, and here she was genuinely pleased that we had the greenlight to proceed perhaps in a different direction. She was not afraid of new information or information that may be counter to what she believed. Rather she was embracing the opportunity to learn more and then follow whatever path we determined through this process. No entrenchment. Only openness and trust.

"I am pulling together the team today. Will have the time commitment, schedule, plan, process, etc. all in place by first thing in the morning."

"Rock on, Tom!"

REFLECTION

One of the biggest differences between a VoC and a focus group is the VoC process uses open- ended questions and allows the 'customer' to drive the direction whereas the focus group tends to hone in on a specific area ... such as benefits in this case. The VoC is a market-in approach to informing decisions, and I believed here we had a wonderful opportunity to truly engage our members and patients in a whole new way. Where rather than us directing them to the answer we wanted, we'd leverage this new approach and open our hearts and minds to new data, new information, new wisdom.

Too often, we "experts" think we know it all and simply "go through the paces" to attain input from those we serve.

The VoC created an opportunity for us to be vulnerable ... and to learn. Yes, a step toward becoming a learning organization in an effort to better meet the needs of those who need us most.

Questions

1. As a healthcare leader, clinician, or staff person, have you used focus groups to leverage a market-in approach to growth or other mission aligned initiatives?
    a. If so, what worked best?
    b. Where were the opportunities to improve the process?
    c. What is the number one recommendation you would make to someone interested in obtaining the input of your staff, patients, families, doctors, nurses, and others?
2. As a healthcare leader, clinician, or staff person, do you believe it is important to listen to the voice of patients and families / doctors and nurses / and others in order to achieve your mission? Why or why not?
    a. How are you currently engaging these people in order to achieve your mission? What is working? Where do you need help?
    b. What is the first thing you would recommend someone do if they were interested in truly engaging patients and families in care improvement?
3. As a clinician or staff person, have you been part of a team where you felt safe, supported, whole, and positioned to do your best?
    a. If so, what key things contributed to such a team?
    b. If not, what barriers existed which prevented such a team culture, and what would you do to change it?
4. As a healthcare leader, clinician, or staff person, as you reflect on Saul and Claire's approach to leadership, are you open to new ideas or entrenched in your own thinking?

Chapter 10

The Team

"Thank you all for your willingness to dedicate your valuable time to this quality improvement project. You each represent a different perspective and thus a different lens in which to better position each of us to honor all those we serve."

"Tracie, you, of course, represent our care management area."

It was the first meeting of the collaborative team I had pulled together for this important project. I was both excited and anxious knowing how much depended on our work together and the potential impact we could make.

Tracie was a recent hire by Saul. A good leader and nurse with excellent credentials. I remember thinking how very much I looked forward to learning more from and about her during this process.

"Frank, you represent our provider network."

I hired Frank to replace me in the provider network leadership role when I moved into the COO position. He was solid if not overtly passionate. I hoped to develop a closer relationship with him during this process.

"Michelle, you are bringing to us the marketing perspective."

Michelle was hired by Claire and tapped to join this cross-functional team. She was a fairly recent college graduate and eager to learn and grow.

"Stephen, you truly represent our military members. I am especially thrilled that you have the time to join us."

"It is my duty to be here representing those we serve and ensuring we stay focused on their real needs."

Stephen's dedication and focus on serving humbles me to this day.

"Esther, as always thrilled to be partnering with you. You represent the relationship we have with the Department of Defense in addition to ensuring we remain true to our mission."

"Like Stephen, and you Tom, the military families and retirees we serve are of utmost importance to me. I must be here."

Having Esther say "and you Tom" in this context truly touched me. And as I held her gaze, I remember a warmth building behind my eyes.

"Thank you, Esther. You being here means a lot and will truly position us to honor these folks."

"Cheryl, so glad you are here. You are representing corporate finance. Thank you for making the time."

Cheryl was another younger member of the team. She is smart and caring and a pleasure to work with. Years later, she will leave the finance area and join the front lines as a dedicated nurse. I would like to think that perhaps this experience helped nudge her in that direction.

"Julie, I have heard many good things about you but have not had the pleasure to meet you in person. Thank you for joining us from the practice side of the house and representing our patients through your lens as a nurse and hands-on caregiver."

"Thank you, Tom. I am excited to learn the Voice of the Customer process and to help any way I can."

"And last but not least," yes, I know, quite a cliché, "Cathy. You will be representing the administrative and support areas of our military program on this team. I always enjoy our collaborations and look forward to another successful outcome."

"Thank you, Tom. I am looking forward to putting to good use the Voice of the Customer process we learned through CQM."

"We have much work to do in a short amount of time, and I know that together and with the voices and requirements we gather from our patients and members, we will learn and improve all we do."

I remember reading in the leadership book "Make it So", which uses Jean-Luc Picard of Star Trek the Next Generation as the role model for effective leading, the importance of focusing on a single mission, the importance of effective communication, the value of teamwork, and how critical it is to be honorable and with high integrity.

And yet what also came to mind for me in this setting and at this time was a story which I believe is from this book but perhaps was actually strictly from the show itself.

Captain Picard and Dr. Beverly Crusher were stranded on a planet together and somehow, they were able to read one another's thoughts. And as I recall it, at one point the doctor asked the captain something to the effect of, "Captain, which direction do we go from here?" To which Jean-Luc replied, "We go to the right." But because Dr. Crusher could read the Captain's mind she was aware that Jean-Luc actually had no idea which way to go but as the leader knew he needed to make a decision and, when he did, to do so with great confidence.

And again, for some reason this scene came to mind for me as my team and I embarked on a new journey together (exploring strange new worlds one might say) using a process some of us have just learned but have never used and others have only heard about. Yes, we had a very strict deadline, but we also had a sole mission and I believed a solid team to "make it so." Could we fail and waste both time and money and do so very publicly (inside and outside of the organization)? Yes. And yet, I didn't believe we would. We had passion. And we had a tool that I believed we could master … together. So even if the odds were stacked against us a bit, I believed in our team and our mission, and that is the confidence I displayed (even if in the back of my mind I too had concerns ala Jean-Luc).

I continued …

"Tell me a Fact and I will Learn. Tell me the Truth and I will Believe. Tell me a Story and it will Remain in my Heart."

(Native American Proverb)

"Together we will be gathering stories from patients and members through the process of collecting the voice of our customers. And these stories (these voices) will be their 'truths' … we will learn from them, we will remember them, and we will improve who we are and what we do because we will believe them."

I took a breath and then ….

"Through the Voice of the Customer process, which we will experientially learn together … so no worries … we will turn these stories into requirements, which we will then prioritize and convert to actionable information in order to evolve and improve the care and the service we provide."

And then over the next three or so hours together, we reviewed and became familiar with the basics of the VoC process and clarified our purpose statement, prior to reviewing the historical data from the previously conducted focus groups, survey data, and information from the growth team 7-step process I had led previously.

Our finalized purpose statement:

> "To determine what is most important to our patients and members by truly listening to understand with our hearts and minds to the voices of our customers in order to better serve, care, and support them on their health and healthcare journey."

NOTE: I am not enamored with the term "customer" in the context of healthcare but chose to remain true to the process (including the terminology) as we proceeded with implementing the VoC for the first time, rather than cloud our focus.

And when we finished our data review ...

"So the answer is ... NETWORK, NETWORK, NETWORK! Right?" I said tongue in cheek.

And of course Frank responded, "Absolutely!"

Before Michelle interjected, "No. It's a new benefit. A new Dental benefit to be exact."

And as we continued our discussion, it became very apparent to me that each of us came into this process with our own biases, pre-conceived notions, and "sure-fire" solutions. And if we were to truly get to the heart of meeting the real needs of those we serve; we truly did need to open our hearts and minds (just as we said in our aim statement).

And together over the next few hours and days and weeks, we also learned:

- We could no longer drive change using strictly a "product-out" approach where we made decisions using internal knowledge only while maintaining a belief system and culture where we believe that our patients and members don't know enough to be helpful and are not "expert" enough to help guide organizational decisions.

- That the voice of our patients and members were, in fact essential, in order to guide our decisions while maintaining our True North.

- And to do this, we learned we needed to hear their voices, their whole stories, and from these stories identify their requirements and, thus, our priorities.

- We needed to engage our patients and members in a whole new way, upfront and as part of our design process. Proactively.

- And to do so, we needed to create safe space and share time with one another and with these folks to develop authentic relationships and trust so that they would be willing to share their voices (their stories), and we would be willing to truly listen and then honor them through our actions.

So yes, on this first day we accomplished a great deal ... and yet still had much further to go.

Later that night …

> *"Patient's harmed. And worse yet … military families hurt. Physician practices are just human factories, and patients are on a conveyor belt. Get them in and out they say. There is no compassion left in healthcare. More tonight on the 6 o'clock news."*

NO! NO! NO!

"Tom, wake up. You are having a nightmare."

Thank God it was only a nightmare. Or was it?

"I hear Tommy stirring. Why don't you and Angus go get him and take him downstairs to play? But be careful not to wake the girls."

Focusing on my boy and my puppy for a little while sounded great to me.

"And put the coffee on too."

"Yes, dear. Anything for you," I joked.

"Angus. Where is my good pup? Let's go get Tommy! Let's go get the boy!"

And after tiptoeing out of our bedroom Angus and I crossed the hallway to Tommy's door.

"Big T," I whispered.

And then, also in a whisper, "Angus, go get the boy."

"Daddy!"

"Big T!"

"Love you, Daddy!"

"I love you! I see you have your Super Boy pajamas on still. Do you want to fly downstairs with Angus and me and play?"

"YEAH!!!!!!!"

Oops. Doc is going to kill me if I wake up the girls, I remember thinking.

"Shhhhhh, Big T. We need to be stealthy. I mean we need to be quiet, so the girls don't wake up."

"They don't want to play with us?"

"It is not that, T. They just need more sleep than us boys today. Perhaps tomorrow they will get up first."

"Okay, Daddy. Can I bring Spidey?"

"Your new Spiderman on his wicked cool motorcycle? Of course! How could we play without Harley-Spidey?!"

"You're funny, Daddy."

"Thanks, T. Now get your cape. Super Boy must have his cape."

"Got it! Can you put it back on for me?"

"You betcha."

Thank God for Velcro, I thought as I nimbly (for a 35-year-old man very early in the morning and in the dark) secured Tommy's red cape full of super powers onto the back of each of his broad shoulders.

"Look at my muscles, Daddy," Tommy said as he did his best double-bicep Arnold pose.

"Wow. Are you kidding me? Did you stick socks in your sleeves? Your muscles are huge. Pythons!"

"Let's go, Daddy!"

"Ok. Angus lead the way. Time to play downstairs."

"YEAH!!!!"

"Tommy, shhhhhhh…"

Doc is always so wise. Playing with Tommy and Angus was exactly what I needed to ease my mind this morning. The relationship, the trust, and the love of a pup and a child (and a bride) can heal almost anything. At least it could on this morning.

REFLECTION

There has been much discussion as to the "appropriate" term for patients in the healthcare system, e.g., patient, customer, consumer, person.

"Customer" (or "consumer" for that matter) is not my preferred term for our patients. And even though I have great respect for Regina Herzlinger (see: Consumer-Driven Healthcare) and others who use these terms, I find the engagement of patients and families in healthcare related decision-making far different than purchasing French Fries from McDonald's. And I see these individuals as more than just purchasers of services. Much more, in fact.

Add to the fact that many (most) patients and families are not well-versed in medical terminology, medical research, care guidelines, standards of care ... (how could they be?)) ... the relationship between a patient and family and the healthcare system is far different than someone who has gone online, researched the latest smart phone, and then journeyed to the closest box store to make a purchase.

Now add to the equation that many times the patient is facing a life or death situation, or a life- altering decision. Many are compromised due to physical pain, emotional stress, and so much more.

Never mind that in the current model of care, although this is changing a bit with high deductible and catastrophic plans, the actual payer of many of the services is not the patient and family at all but a third party be it Medicare, Medicaid, or an insurance carrier.

No, a patient is not a customer or a consumer. A patient is a patient. A patient is a person. And we in the healthcare system must develop an entirely different kind of relationship with these people than we would with a purchaser of French fries or smart phones.

Questions

1. As a healthcare leader, clinician, or staff person, how have you remained open (heart and mind) to new ideas? Please share a story.
    a. What tools do you use to engage cross-functional teams?
    b. What if any downsides have you experienced of using cross-functional teams to achieve a goal?
    c. How have you overcome these challenges?
2. As a healthcare leader, clinician, staff person, patient, or family member, how do you manage stress?
    a. How do you process any negative thoughts that creep into your mind?
    b. How do you remain present?
    c. How do you ensure a balanced life?

Chapter 11

Back to the VoC

"Good morning, Team."

"Good morning, Tom."

"Where is Stephen?"

"Oh, I have been here [voice from the kitchen]. Just making a new pot of coffee for everyone."

God, I love him.

"Where do we go from here, Tom?"

"Perfect question, Esther."

For the next couple of hours, we reviewed and discussed each stage and step of our process while mindfully reflecting on our mission.

We also specifically discussed both network development and benefit offerings noting that much data points to one or both of these solutions and that we must both be open to these data while also being open to new information and new learnings.

"Tom, I know you trust this process. And I know I trust you. We trust you. Let's really learn what will best meet our patients' and members' needs … from our patients and members."

Although this was exactly what any leader would want to hear, thinking about my restless night this sentiment truly touched my heart. Especially coming from Esther.

"Thank you, Esther. That is exactly right. Together we are going to learn from these folks, from their viewpoint, from their lens, and then honor them by improving what we do based on their wisdom."

And then after scanning the room …

"Now, and most importantly at this juncture … is there more coffee?"

Late that afternoon, and mentally exhausted after many more hours of collaborative effort, we confirmed all of our accomplishments of the day, including: completing our customer profile matrix, developing an interview guide, confirming our interview approach, practicing our interview and transcribing skills, and more. I turned to my team …

"I cannot imagine what you have waiting for you in your emails and voicemails. What work is piling up for you. I so appreciate all you are bringing to the table each day. Let's call it a day. Have a wonderful evening. We will be back at this at 10am the day after tomorrow."

I had built in a day for folks to try to catch up on some of the other work they were responsible for.

"Thank you, Team."

And even later that evening after I had caught up on some of my other work, I phoned Doc from the car.

"Doc?"

"You sound so tired. Don't talk. Just come home to me."

REFLECTION

With the fact that we all learn differently at top of mind ... I crafted the poem Painfully Standing Tall for all those people feeling alone and marginalized as they try to turn the tide and heal the broken healthcare system.

PAINFULLY STANDING TALL

ALONE IN HUMANITY
HARM FINDING ALL
POWER WIELDING PARITY
PAINFULLY STANDING TALL

QUESTIONING IF TO JOIN THE BASE
IS IT POSSIBLE TO WIN THIS RACE
WITH A SHADOW COVERED FACE
AND ONE'S HEART IN FULL DISGRACE

STAYING THE COURSE WITH THE FEW
SO MUCH SURELY STILL ASKEW
OWE IT TO THE HARMED AND THE HURTING
REGRETS BE DAMNED, THERE IS NO DIVERTING

FOLLOW? YOU CANNOT DO
SERVE AND LEAD YOU MUST
HELPING OTHERS LONG OVERDUE
TOGETHER WE WILL TRUST

TIME TO ARISE
YOUR MIND AND YOUR HEART
AS MANY DESPISE
WE ALL DO OUR PART

VULNERABLE AND OPEN
FACING POWERS THAT BE

IN ACTION NOT HOPING OF SERVICE TO THEE

Please know … you are not alone.

There are many amazing, smart, heart-centered, caring people inside and outside of the healthcare system who share your passion, your fear, your highs, and your lows … all striving to help others and improve the system for all.

Don't be discouraged. Have faith. And if you ever need a place to turn … just let me know.

There are many flames of goodness all around us … together we can fan them (support one another) and benefit many.

Questions

1. As a healthcare leader or clinician, how do you ensure your team feels valued?
    a. Is authentically caring about (loving) your team important to you? Why? Why not?
    b. Can a team be successful without feeling valued?
2. As a team member, what are the top three things that best position you for success?
3. As a healthcare leader, clinician, or staff person, how has fear held you back from achieving a goal?
    a. What have you learned from this?
    b. How do you manage your fear now?
    c. How do you assist your team to manage its fears?

Chapter 12

Mrs. Jones

With our tools created and our process confirmed, we were now ready to truly listen to our "customers."

"We have a great opportunity here. Over the next few days, we will be connecting with those who under normal circumstances many of us would never meet during the course of our normal workday. And as we engage these folks, I believe we will be hearing things we never could expect. I am so encouraged by what we have done to date and so very much look forward to coming back together to share the voices we have heard … the stories we will have listened to … and learn. Learn what we are doing right, learn what we are doing wrong, learn where we have systems in which we need to improve, and learn where we need to rethink what we do and why we do it."

"Tom, are you ready to head out. Our first interview is in an hour with Linda Jones, a 64-year-old, female, existing member and patient, married to a retired military officer, living in Maine (down in the Cape Ellis area), who says she is happy with our program."

"Excellent, Michelle. I just need to grab my briefcase and a cup of coffee and then I will be all set to go."

"I think this is a good discussion to begin with. Should be positive."

"We shall see, Michelle. We shall see. Remember open heart and mind."

The day was gorgeous. The sun still low in the sky but bright and casting shadows. And as we walked to my car, the shadows from the sun and trees cast along the ground reminded me of our own shadows and of our own projections.

The ride to Camp Ellis from Portland was just under 40 minutes (approximately 25 miles). And by the time we arrived at Mrs. Jones' house, I believe both Michelle and I had a combination of both butterflies and confidence in what we were doing.

"Hi, Mrs. Jones?"

"Yes. I am Mrs. Jones."

"My name is Tom Dahlborg and this is Michelle St. Onge. I believe you were expecting us?"

"Oh yes. I have been looking forward to meeting with you and talking about the experiences of my husband and me with the military healthcare program. Come in. Come in."

Mrs. Jones' home was on Route 9. In fact, her front door was literally less than ten feet from the road itself.

Her home with its grey shingles and bright red trim reminded me of the homes we would see on Cape Cod, where I spent much of my youth.

"What a beautiful place, Mrs. Jones." I said.

"Please call me, Linda."

"Okay, Linda."

"Let's talk out in the three-season room. Would either of you like some tea or water?"

"Michelle?"

"Some water would be wonderful."

"Yes, Linda, some water would be much appreciated."

"Well, you two get comfortable and set up as you need. I will be right back."

A few moments later …

"Here are your waters." And then, while looking at a cozy light blue with beige flowers padded rocking chair, "And you left me my favorite seat. Perfect. Just perfect," Mrs. Jones said with a smile.

"Mrs. Jones, I mean, Linda, thank you for allowing Michelle and me to meet with you today. We do so appreciate your willingness to share with us."

"Oh, I have much to say, young man."

"Linda, we were planning on about an hour – is that still okay?"

"Oh yes, Michelle, I have all day to share."

"And as a reminder, this is not a sales call. We are not here to sell anything."

"We will see about that."

Linda was a blend of both serious and funny.

"The purpose of our discussion today is to help us to better understand the expectations and requirements of members in our health plan and patients who receive care at our health centers"

"So I am a focus group of one," Linda laughed as she rocked in her chair while sipping her fruity tea. Which I am guessing is a berry blend based on the sweet smell arising and swirling in my direction from the pale green teacup she holds precariously in her hands.

And, of course, what came to mind for me was my own grandmother's tea cups and our afternoon teas together watching Jack Nicklaus and Tom Watson play the back nine or perhaps when we would watch Mr. "Wunnerful" himself, Lawrence Welk, together on her color TV.

Focus Tom. Focus, I reminded myself.

"Do you have any questions before we begin?"

"I sure do," Linda says with a big smile, "Are you two sure you don't want any tea? It is delicious."

And as both Michelle and I say together, "Yes. Actually, that would be wonderful," I think about how being here in this place at this time and with this team in service to others is a dream come true.

After delivering our hot tea in two beautiful tea cups, Linda sat back down and looked from Michelle to me and then said, "Okay, you both have your tea, we are all comfortable, and we have a purpose. I believe we are ready to begin."

"Wow, Linda, clearly you should be leading this discussion."

"Well, this is what happens when you are married to a military officer for so many years. And quite frankly, when you have also led as many people and organizations as I have throughout my career. You learn to set the stage, focus, and get things done."

"Linda, would you please describe to us an experience when you or a loved one needed health care services? Please simply tell us a story."

"Oh, I love stories."

And then after a brief pause ...

"Well, my husband, Mike, isn't doing very well. He has stomach issues. His heart isn't good. He has smoked for years and has tried to quit many, many times. He was active duty for 30 years or so. Saw a lot. Much he doesn't tell me. He always tries to protect me. Just like he always tried to protect his men. He is a stoic man, so I don't always know how bad or good he is doing. I get nervous. Very nervous. And I want to protect him."

Breathe, Tom. Breathe, I silently reminded myself as I listened intently as Linda continued her story of love and mission, of honor and sacrifice.

"... I bring Mike to see his doctor in Portland quite often. We usually see Dr. Black but not always," Linda continued prior to taking a breath and looking up toward the ceiling. "I am not sure why we don't always see Dr. Black. No one tells us. I think I will ask next time. You know, it would just be nice to know," Linda says as she places her hand on my knee and looks deeply into my eyes.

"Do you think they will tell me, Tom?"

"I think they should tell you, Linda. And if they don't, I want to know."

"That would be really great. Mike won't say anything. I guess it is my turn to step up like he always has."

Linda leaned back and was then quiet for a bit as she rocked in her chair and sipped her tea. Clearly a good opportunity for Michelle and me to do the same, I thought.

"You people need to remember something, Tom."

"Yes?"

"Tell me, do you all conduct patient satisfaction surveys?"

"We sure do."

"Now remember, I have worked for a very long time. I am clued in."

"Tell me more."

"I bet the numbers look pretty good. Especially for your military program. True?"

Hmmmm ... what is she getting at? I thought prior to responding based on my learnings, "I believe a score on a good tool conducted the correct way (which we can discuss because I bet I would learn a great deal from you) of anything less than 99% in any category is not good enough. Only at that level have we truly done our job, honored our mission, and created an environment for loyalty."

I actually almost stopped myself from saying loyalty because based on my interactions with the military folks I worked with up to this point they are loyal beyond many (most) non-military personnel I know. And perhaps to their own detriment in some cases.

"That said, Linda, we have many scores into the mid-90's for our military program and, yes, they tend to be touted as quite positive."

"So let me tell you something, Tom."

Linda then inched up to the edge of her rocking chair and took both of my hands into hers.

"Military men like my Mike," I now saw tears in Linda's eyes as she struggled to continue, "These men (and women) are trained to by loyal … and you just said loyalty."

Darn it, I thought, *I know better.*

"These men and women are trained to be loyal. They are trained to overcome. They are trained to not complain. They are trained to follow orders. They are good men and women. And they are well-trained and honorable."

Linda stopped and took a deep breath.

"Tom, your real scores could be in the 60's and they would be loyal. They could (and quite possibly are) being harmed and they would be loyal. Your mid-90's are a misnomer because they do not readily complain. No. They follow orders."

She then sat back and took another deep breath, "Tom. Don't take advantage of their loyalty."

Linda shifted once again in her chair and then stared directly into my soul, "In your role, it is your responsibility. It is your duty. Tell me you will not allow my Mike to be taken advantage of. Tell me you will not allow my Mike's loyalty to lead to his harm."

It was amazing to me. Linda was saying this, and yet I didn't feel anger coming from her. What I felt was a deep love. A deep love that she had for her husband and for all those in service.

"Tom?"

"Linda, we are here for that very reason. We can do better. We want to do better. And we … and I need your help."

Linda continued to hold my hands.

"I believe we understand each other. I believe we both want the same thing." And then looking even deeper still into my eyes (my heart), "And Tom, in my heart, I trust you."

Breathe, Tom. Breathe, I reminded myself once again.

"I hope Michelle is getting all this," I thought as I turned to her and saw a single tear rolling slowly down her cheek.

"Thank you, Linda," I whispered as we all regrouped and readjusted ourselves in our respective seats.

"Now that we are clear, I want to tell you a story from a recent visit."

"Perfect."

"I brought Mike back to Portland to see Dr. Black again. I think this was just last week but perhaps the week before. He wasn't feeling well, and I think his sugars were off. But of course," she winked, "He wouldn't tell me."

"We arrived and stood in line for quite some time to check in. I could tell Mike's legs were bothering him as he shifted his weight from one leg to the other and then back again … but he didn't complain."

Linda paused and looked directly into my eyes again and said, "See what I mean?"

And then continued, "I'll admit, I was getting quite tired too. Not as young as I used to be. But, oh well. When we did eventually get to the front of the line, we checked in and were told to go to the 3rd floor to see Dr. Black."

"So you saw Dr. Black?" I couldn't help myself. I needed to ask.

"Now, Tom, who is telling this story?" came Linda's response.

And I of course thought, *She is my Nana.*

"So we get to the 3rd floor and sit down to wait. And that wasn't so bad." And then with a bit of a chuckle, "You have very good magazines, don't you know?"

"I have noticed that. Especially if you like sailing," I responded.

"Yes! Yes, sailing. We used to love to go out on our boat. Do you sail?"

"Ugh," I thought, based on my own checkered past with boats. So, I just said, "I know many who love to do so."

"Well, if we have time we should talk about sailing. That would be lovely."

And then after a brief pause …

"Anyway, we didn't wait too long before a very lovely nurse came out and said that the doctor would see us now."

Of course, after my 'scolding' I didn't ask which doctor.

"And Tom, it wasn't our doctor. It wasn't Dr. Black. It was another covering doctor. I was so disappointed. And so was Mike, but of course, he didn't say so. But you know what?"

"Tell me, Linda."

"I said so. I told the nurse that we booked our appointment with Dr. Black intentionally and that is who we were told we would see."

"You did? What was the response?"

"Well, clearly Mike wasn't pleased I spoke up. But it was important to me. Dr. Black knows Mike. He knows the challenges Mike has faced, be it his many physical challenges or," and she then whispered, "some mental and emotional challenges he is also facing. Dr. Black knows Mike. We had a plan. We were going to see Dr. Black. We were going to discuss X, Y, and Z, and we were going to follow orders. Tom," and again Linda leaned forward and grabbed my hands, "how is a doctor who has never seen Mike going to know what is best for my Mike? Tell me. Tell me, Tom?"

But before I could answer …

"The appointment was actually okay. We didn't get too deep into anything, and we avoided discussing the mental and emotional health challenges, which I think Mike was embarrassed to share with someone he didn't know anyway, but we will get to that next time we see Dr. Black. But most important on our list that day was to get a couple of prescription refills, and we got those. So overall we did okay."

Linda then sat back in her chair again.

"So Tom, if Mike was completing a patient satisfaction survey on this day, he would have given good scores. But do you see the issues? You do see that his scoring would only reflect let's say, one reality. And it would miss greatly in another. Get it?"

But before I could respond Linda again continued, "You will fix this. I know you will."

"Please tell me more, Linda."

"Only after you and Michelle have some more tea and a couple of homemade pepparkakor cookies."

She is my Nana! I thought once again. And then, "Deal" both Michelle and I said with a smile.

"Well come join me around my kitchen table and we will break bread, or cookies I should say, enjoy some more tea, and continue our discussion."

I cannot wait to learn more, I thought as I pick up my teacup and followed Linda and Michelle.

"Do you have more time than the allotted hour? I think we are going to need it."

I, of course, decide there is no way I was leaving here until Linda has said all she needs to say. It is my duty and I intend to honor her voice and her story. Nothing is more important at this time. Everything else can be rescheduled.

"We are here for you, Linda. If our sharing together requires more than an hour, so be it. As long as you are comfortable with that."

"Wonderful, Tom. Just wonderful. Together, we are going to make a big difference."

I was going to say that, I remember thinking.

"Yes. Yes, we will," I respond with more conviction than I anticipated. Perhaps my concerns were waning as Linda tells her story, and, perhaps, for the first time, her story is truly heard.

"Tom, you don't know how much you and Michelle visiting with me means to me. And to Mike."

Actually, perhaps I do. At least just a little.

"And you know what? Between you two visiting me, sitting with me, and listening to me," and with a tear in her eye, "I feel a little better already. And I know Mike will too."

The pepparkakors were amazing. And it was nice not to get scolded for dunking mine into my hot tea.

"You're a dunker, Tom?" Linda inquired through that loving grin of hers.

"Oh yes. All my life. I hope that is okay."

"Oh yes, Tom. Mike is too. You keep on dunking, and I'll just get you a second napkin just in case."

I laugh as I think about the pepparkakors my Nana would make and how we would joke that my Grandpa would need a bib. I guess it is my turn. But for now, a second napkin will have to do.

After a couple of more cookies and getting to know Linda more, Michelle appropriately redirected us back to our purpose, "Linda, you were going to tell us more about your visit and your prescriptions I believe."

"Oh yes. Oh yes. Sorry about that."

"No need to be sorry whatsoever. Getting to know you, and through you, Mike, is as important as anything else we are meant to do today."

"Okay. Let me see."

And with that Linda this time sits back in her oak kitchen chair and continues …

"Yes. Initially I had thought Mike was okay with not discussing his mental health challenges. But in fact, he wasn't, and I will tell you it began to show later that evening. But at the time he clearly was happy to not be asked by a doctor he did not know, but who was nice enough even though apparently rushed."

Linda became quiet for a few moments as she again leaned forward with her elbows on the kitchen table and pointed at me with her pale slender fingers.

"Tom, we really don't have much to compare things too. Mike had been in the service for a long, long time, and he has been fighting some demons more recently. But I want you to know …"

She paused what seemed like a very long time, and I could see we were both breathing quite deeply.

"… talking to Dr. Black about some mental and emotional health concerns helps a bit. But you know, Dr. Black is not trained in that area. Yes, he is attentive and listens for as long as he can, and that does help, but eventually Mike is referred to someone else."

Another long pause.

"And that doctor, or I should say, those doctors, sometimes a psychiatrist, sometimes a psychologist, etc., they keep changing too. (You all refer to them as Mike's care team but in reality, there is no team. Just ever-changing parts.) And at each subsequent visit, not knowing Mike except for what they read, and not having had a, oh what do you call it, a 'warm handoff' perhaps, they expect Mike to tell his story again and again."

And now Linda is standing as she leans on the kitchen table.

"That is wrong you two. It is unfair, it is unhelpful, it is painful, and it is painful to watch. It is just plain wrong. There is no continuity. There may be caring, but that is buried well below the broken system."

And with tears now rolling down her cheeks … "Mike has been hurt enough. Why should the healthcare system, which was built to supposedly take care of him, hurt him more? Can you answer that for me?"

Linda's face had now lost the radiance it had when we first met about an hour ago. The glow is gone. Now her face shows the etchings from the battles she faces each day loving and supporting her husband and trying to navigate the broken healthcare system.

"It shouldn't harm, Linda. The healthcare system should not harm anyone, let alone a soldier and his family," I whispered. "I am so sorry."

I pause to allow Linda the time to resituate in her chair.

And as I pause Michelle rightfully shares, "We are also sorry to cause you any pain today as we have this conversation. We can stop at any time."

"Oh Deary, don't mind my tears. You two are already helping me heal. And together we will help Mike heal."

And then …

"Tom, clearly you have a special team. And I can tell you both care. I can feel it." She paused and takes a sip of her tea. "Thank you for being here with me. Please know it really does mean so much. Even if you hear me vent a bit and witness a shed tear or two."

We all sat back in our chairs and enjoyed more of our cookies and fruit tea. Yes, with me dunking all the while.

And as we do, I continue to remember thinking how even more determined I am now. How I know the goodness within our organization. And also know that along with most (possibly all) healthcare systems, at least in the United States, productivity is becoming even more the god. 'Churn the RVUs (aka relative value units), get even more patients in and out of the office, turf any mental health issues, and leverage technology, ancillary services and the higher reimbursement for more invasive procedures to maximize revenue.' Yes, even more determined now that I am truly seeing the impact of the reality of the system. Yes, even with value-based purchasing, productivity remains king.

And as I ate my cookies and sipped my tea, out of nowhere Michael Jordan's quote came to me, "I know fear is an obstacle for some people, but it is an illusion to me. Failure always made me try harder next time." And that gave me some comfort.

"Linda …" I then began to say but she cut me off.

"Before I forget, I want to tell you about getting the prescriptions I refilled for Mike at your pharmacy the day of his appointment."

Yes, we had our own pharmacy at our Portland site.

"As I was saying, Mike seemed okay at the time not talking about any mental health stuff with the new doctor." And then Linda turned directly to me, "Again, he was very nice. Just new. And apparently very rushed."

"Anyway, I could tell Mike was tired, and I will be honest, I was tired too, don't you know," Linda continued with a smile. And I could see the radiance reemerge in her face as her blue eyes sparkled again.

She continued, "So when we got off the elevator, I told him, 'Mike, you sit down and I will go stand in line for your prescriptions.' There was quite a line at the time, but Mike needed his scripts, and I was going to stand there as long as it took."

"Yes, I know. It can get very busy for sure," Michelle responded empathetically.

"Mike knows to follow orders," Linda said as she began to laugh heartily, "And especially from me!"

Oh, how I loved seeing and hearing this beautiful woman laugh and, of course, Michelle and I laughed too. Perhaps too soon though.

And after she caught her breath the smile was again gone from her face.

"So I got in line. And although there was another window to the pharmacy, that one was not open, so I stood behind seven or eight other people and waited my turn."

"How long was your wait?"

"Oh, not too long, Michelle."

"Is that 'not too long' from the perspective of a dutiful soldier's wife?" I asked.

"Oh you caught me, Tom." Linda responded with a smirk as she pointed at me. "You caught me. You are right. Like I said, trained to follow orders and not complain."

After taking another sip of tea, Linda did share with us that she waited over forty minutes in the line for her husband's prescription refills while being very tired, worrying about Mike not having his mental health items discussed, and as her legs ached.

And as she did, my heart ached.

"But I don't want this to be about me."

"Linda, we are here to serve all of our members and patients and their families. That means you too. And by learning from you, we can help others," Michelle responded.

Linda paused for a bit, looking as if she was debating whether to share more or not, and then eventually said, "Well. Do you know what the pharmacist said to me when I finally got to the open window?"

With Michael Jordan's words still echoing in my ears I was ready. *Tell us, Linda. Tell us exactly what was said*, I thought to myself as I prepared to respond. But she beat me to it.

"Well, let me tell you."

Linda's smile was still nowhere to be seen.

"When I handed the two prescription refills to the pharmacist I said to him, 'My husband's stomach has been bothering him for a long time and he finds that having 'coated' tablets," Linda stopped for a moment and looked from Michelle to me, "I didn't know what else to call them," she then continued, "I said to him, 'having 'coated' tablets would be best because the non-coated tablets upset his stomach."

Linda paused again. And again, I could see tears well up in her eyes as she leaned back in her chair and placed one of her delicate hands to her shoulder and the other up toward her neck as if she were protecting herself from an expected blow.

And as she looked to the floor she said as her voice began to tremble, "He said," and then her voice broke, "No, he screamed so everyone around could hear," and as she continued her voice got softer, "he screamed, 'Who the Hell do you think you are?! Who!? I can't get that for you! How the hell do you think I can get them just for you?'"

My heart pounded as my stomach became hollow. This smart, kind, loving, supportive, amazing woman ... who reminded me so of my Nana, was being harmed by the system I supported. By the system we created.

My head and heart began to battle internally, "NO! How could this be? It is not possible." And I could feel my defenses rising I must admit.

But eventually both my head and heart won and the unexpressed defensiveness, 'Thank God unexpressed,' was pushed aside as my heart and mind opened further.

Linda sat for a long while not moving, just staring at the floor as I projected that she was reliving being yelled at in front of many as she tried to get two prescriptions refilled while protecting her husband from more harm. I also projected how she must have felt with her dignity (a dignity she carried so very well with her warm smile and big heart married to her tenacity and love for her husband) being stripped away publicly.

"Tom," Linda finally said (so low I had to lean over the table to hear her).

"Yes."

"I simply wanted to take care of my husband the way he has always taken care of me. To take care of him the way he always took care of his men. To take care of ..."

She began to trail off, so I simply waited.

"I simply wanted to take care of him the way I would want someone to take care of ..."

Again, quiet as Linda's hand moved from her shoulder to the table and eventually to mine.

"The way I would want someone to take care of me," she cried.

I was wrong.

No matter how much the health system tried to take it ... this amazing woman's dignity was never lost.

REFLECTION

Even now, fifteen years later, there is much in the news about the horrors of the healthcare system for our military folks.

From infection rates to improperly done procedures:

> *"Half of the military's largest hospitals performed worse than established benchmarks in categories such as infections or improperly done procedures, according to a review from the American College of Surgeons. The college compared each hospital with an expected rate of complications based on the procedures it performed and what kinds of patients it served from July 2012 to June 2013."*
>
> *Sources: Department of Defense, American College of Surgeons.*

To wait times leading to patient harm and death:

> *"'Phoenix is just the tip of the iceberg,' Selnick said, referring to last week's announcement that VA Secretary Eric Shinseki had placed three Phoenix veterans' hospital officials on administrative leave after several former employees alleged that as many as 40 patients may have died as a result of treatment delays. Whistle-blowers also claimed that a secret list of patients waiting for appointments had been maintained to conceal how long it took for patients to be treated."*
> *Source: Modern Healthcare, Pattern of problems with Veterans Affairs healthcare system, Rachel Landen | May 7, 2014*

This is unacceptable treatment for any patient and family. This is unacceptable for military patients and families. This is not healthcare. And this is nowhere close to healthCARING.

Through our VoC, we learned a great deal about the challenges facing military retirees and dependents within our system. And that was almost 20 years ago.

What is occurring today remains unacceptable and unconscionable.

Questions

1. As a healthcare leader, clinician, staff person, patient or family member, please share a story of your experience with military healthcare.
   a. Please shine a light on the goodness within the system so that we may fan these flames of good.
   b. Or share a different experience, an experience which will open our eyes to those places where we can improve and make a difference.
   c. And/or share other thoughts and perspectives in an effort to productively move us forward to benefit those that we serve.
2. As a healthcare leader, clinician, or staff person, are you using patient satisfaction scores to assess patient experience and satisfaction?
   a. If so, how are you accounting for cultural, generational, and other differences such as explained by Linda relative to military personnel, in how surveys are responded to and the meanings?
   b. How have you assessed the story behind the satisfaction scores?
3. Is your organization truly trying to understand the survey outcomes data or rather simply using them to tout a number?
4. What are the unintended consequences of a reliance on satisfaction scores and how you are managing them?

Chapter 13

Voices of Our Customers

About a week later, after our team had completed all of our interviews, we came back together.

"Quite a week," Cheryl began, as we were gathering around the conference room table each with our coffee or tea and perhaps a muffin in hand.

"Transformative," Tracie interjected.

"We thought so too," came from Michelle.

"In many ways, I am proud of what we do. I am also a bit discouraged too," Frank shared.

"These interviews gave me a whole new look at what we do," Cathy continued the sharing.

"And who we do it with and who we do it for," I added.

"Yes, exactly. Did you look into the eyes of these folks? Did you experience …"

Experience! I thought.

Julie continued "… their sincerity? Their desire to help?"

"Yes! That is our military folk," Esther said with great (and appropriate) pride.

"And they were not all military. Remember some were non-military patients," Stephen said, and then after a breath or two and with his voice trailing off just a bit, "And still I noticed many of the same things."

For the next twenty minutes or so, we focused first on our community (our team). We checked in as to how and what we were feeling and how or if we needed supports of our own. We then shared our gut reactions and our feelings associated with the process prior to moving onto discussions specific to each of our encounters with these patients and members … these people.

And as we did so, I made sure I looked around the table and visually connected with each member of our team. And yes, I did see a bit of discouragement, at least initially, but as we continued as a group, as a team, I saw and felt a different energy. An energy change. And the more we shared as a team, a team that became close through this experience over the past week or so, I witnessed this new energy grow. In fact, I saw a wave of energy circling the table like a literal *wave* around a sports arena as encouragement and 'we cannot fail' and 'we owe it to them' took hold and replaced any discouragement.

And only at this point did I know we were ready to share the voices we heard. And over the next four hours those voices filled the room.

"Because the tests that were run on me were negative, I had to literally get on my hands and knees and beg for follow-up because nobody believed me when I said I was still in pain."

And …

"My wife called the doctor's when she had a temperature of 102 degrees. She was told they would call back. Three hours later, they had not. I called again. At that point, my wife's temperature was 104 degrees. I was told they would get back to me because no appointments were available. I then got in my car and drove my wife to the doctor's. The doctor finally saw her when her temperature was at 105. The doctor called 911 and my wife ended up in the hospital for a week. I almost lost her."

And then Cathy added, "And he cried. And so did I," as a tear rolled down her cheek.

After many more of these voices were heard, I addressed my team again, "This is why we are here. We have challenges before us. And together and with our members and patients, we will make things better. This is clearly hard AND it is important that we listen to these voices and truly hear them as we work to improve what we do each day. And when we do, then and only then will we know we truly honored these voices and our patients. Now let's take a break, grab some sandwiches, get a drink of water or soda, and come back together in 20 minutes."

"Good timing," Frank and Cheryl said in unison as we all rose to indulge in the Anania delicacies and catch our breath.

Perhaps this 'breathing' stuff has something to it?

After lunch we came back together.

And Cathy began, "Team, I am so sorry for crying earlier."

"Oh, please don't be," Julie responded as did the others.

"I am actually quite pleased that we have each had an experience that touched us so deeply. I know I am forever changed by my personal encounters," Julie continued.

"I was very sick," another voice was being shared by Tracie, "I waited as long as I could, until I was on my deathbed." Tracie then looked up from her post it notes and gazed into each of our eyes, "He did not want to burden us. This patient of ours, this member of ours, did not want to burden the healthcare system, so he waited rather than calling back after being told there were no appointments available for him and not being provided with any other options." Tracie then paused and took a deep breath of her own before repeating, but this time in a whisper, "He did not want to burden us."

"He did not want to burden us? No way. This stops with us. We are going to fix this," Esther, practically standing, said with the command of her military training.

Yes! I thought as others chimed in.

"Tom, I know we have a process, and a good one, but we need solutions … now," Frank added.

"I swear I will do all I can to ensure the system gets fixed so our members, military or not, never feel this way again," came from Stephen.

And universally, the energy and the sentiment remained focused where it needed to be.

"Together we will make a difference. Together we will turn these voices into solutions and with our patients and members, we will fix this brokenness." And then, after an unintentional dramatic pause, as I took a breath, I continued, "Frank, I am with you. We need to fix this. And we need to fix it quickly. And we will do so through the process to ensure we do what is most impactful and not simply what might feel good. And Stephen, I love your passion, and everyone's passion. We cannot own another's feelings, but we can fix systems. And we will …"

"I know, Tom. I know. But these are my brothers and sisters."

"And we will fix this. For them," I responded to Stephen and then turned to Tracie, "Tracie, please continue."

Tracie began again, "He continued, 'When I was on my deathbed I called again and was offered an appointment in a week and I responded,'" Tracie caught her breath, "'I responded that I would be dead by then and that she better find something sooner.'" Tracie then looked up at us all, "Believe it or not, Team, he actually felt guilty for saying that to the individual making the appointments. He felt guilty for saying that to us."

"Those are the types of members we have. And especially our retired military folk," Esther said with conviction and again with pride. "And that is why our member and patient satisfaction scores must be looked at far differently than say a 'typical' health plan or medical site. Our 90% satisfaction equates to another plan's 70%, I would think."

"Esther, one of the people, who Tom and I met with, is a retired professional woman married to a military officer, and she said the same type of thing."

"It is so true, Michelle. So very true," Esther responded.

"Another takeaway for all of us," I noted, "As we continue on this journey. And in and of itself, such a nugget of wisdom that without this process I would never have known. Frank, would you please make note of this (the limitations of patient satisfaction scores) in the 'parking lot.'"

> Note: The 'parking lot' is for us this day a flip chart where key nuggets of wisdom that may not be 100% aligned with our directive can be gathered in order to not be lost in order to be followed up upon later.

Over the next four hours, we shared more stories, ensured we understood what each was telling us and began to group them into categories (themes).

Some of the stories were truly 'cringe worthy' and others were still serious but more operational with less of a 'tug on the heart' impact.

We heard:

> "I had hoped I could see the doctor I selected. Instead, he retired, and I don't know what happened to the next two. Nobody told me."

> "Turnover of doctors is a negative. I have had five or six in ten years. They come and go unfortunately. I have had the same doctor for the last two years. My fingers are crossed."

> "Dr. Black is too busy to see us. We were forced to select a new doctor, Dr. Brooks. Dr. Brooks spent time with us and listened to us. Then you had to go and get rid of her because she was too slow."

We also heard: "I have been told that my tumor is inoperable, but you won't let me seek out other treatment options. You don't care if I live or die."

And as we continued our process of gathering, defining, sorting and learning together I could see some dismay again but also, with great kudos to the team, more of what I saw was passion. A passion to fan the flames of what was working well and a passion to fix the broken.

"These voices are so difficult to hear, but like we said earlier, we must. We owe it to our members and patients. We owe it to ourselves."

"Well said, Cheryl. And I agree 100%. I had no idea. Working in Network Development I knew about access issues due to the need to expand networks, but the doctor turnover, the rules our patients are dealing with, and the impact on their very lives," Frank paused as he peered out the window at the sun shining onto Casco Bay and then continued very softly, "I had no idea. I can't imagine my parents or my grandparents having to deal with these barriers to care. I can't imagine."

"I agree," Michelle chimed in. "I 'knew' coming into this that the solution was a benefit solution." She then chuckled a bit and looked at Frank, "Being in marketing what did you expect?"

"I know what you mean," Frank responded acknowledging again his Network Development lens (or as I like to say, probably too often, "when you have a hammer everything looks like a nail").

"But it is not," Michelle continued, "a benefit issue." Drawing a deep breath, she finished her thought with, "This is much more profound."

"A benefit solution would be a technical fix where what we are hearing, seeing, feeling and learning is that some of these voices are actually highlighting challenges that require adaptive solutions." After a scan of the room to see if folks were following, I continued, "Yes, there are some technical fixes we can make and they will make a difference and have an impact with phone systems and processes, for example, but it is becoming more and more apparent that we will need adaptive solutions for these larger issues." I paused again as I considered whether I have now gotten ahead of myself.

And, after what appeared to be a dramatic pause for affect but was actually simply me collecting my thoughts, I continued, "With that said, let's continue. Julie?"

Julie shared the following patient voice, "I had just had a wonderful visit with my doctor. He is so nice and so attentive. I was so happy, but then when I told the person at the checkout desk that I had had such a nice visit with my doctor and that I think that he is just wonderful, she responded to me with a glare and said, 'Your doctor is an idiot. He doesn't know anything.'"

"My god. Why? Why would someone …," Cathy said under her breath but loud enough for folks close to her to hear.

"Could be lots of reasons," Cheryl responded. Then, "I think that voice segues right into this one. May I?"

"Absolutely," I responded.

"One of your pharmacy techs was furious with you all and was saying very loudly to her co-worker, and so that all of us patients could hear, 'I am going to leave this place as soon as I can'. And she was saying this while she was filling medicine bottles left and right. Needless to say, I checked my prescription very carefully that night to ensure there was no mistake."

And before anyone could react Frank spoke up, "I have another voice in this area I believe." And then after sorting through his post-it notes, he shared the following, "I see Dr. Iuvenis who is covering for Dr. Black. He tells me he is going to change my allergy meds. (Yes, the ones that Dr. Black and I spent so long getting right). He didn't tell me why. He didn't even ask me. He just told me that he knows best."

"What is going on here?"

"I don't know, Esther. I don't know. But we will figure it out," Tracie said as she put her hand on Esther's shoulder.

"Why do you think doctors and nurses and staff would behave like this?"

"I am not sure, Frank," came Tracie's response. "I wonder if they are burnt out? I wonder if these behaviors are manifesting because the system we have created has abused them and, if so, to what degree and, of course, what we can do about it? I have seen nurses act out in hospitals after being mistreated for so long. Same with physicians coming out of medical school. Some act out, some harm themselves, some even worse. Perhaps it is the same here? And again, to what extent? But don't get me wrong, there is no excuse for these behaviors."

"Such an important point, Tracie. And in quality improvement speak 'you get the outcome the system is designed to achieve.' Definitely another focus area for us to keep in mind as we continue ... 'how do we ensure all stakeholders throughout the system are whole and healthy to ensure they (we) are all best positioned to truly care for one another?'" I responded.

It was getting late at this point, and we had now surpassed five and a half hours.

"Are you okay, Tracie?"

"Oh yes, Tom. I think someone must have moved the doorway over the last few hours."

Tracie had gotten up to get a glass of water and as she was about to enter the kitchen (which is just off of the conference room) bashed her shoulder into the door jamb.

"Are you sure? I will get you some ice," Stephen chimed in as he made his way out of the conference room and through the doorway, which actually had not moved.

"We are all getting tired. How would you like to stop for now and finish this portion of our process tomorrow?" I inquired.

"I don't know about anyone else, but I would like to complete this stage. My shoulder is fine. And as for more tiredness, I believe I smell some more coffee brewing, so I will be fine momentarily."

"Thank you, Tracie. And please do whatever you need to do for your shoulder. Others?" I asked as I scanned the room.

"It would be great to have all the voices compiled and understood and sorted before we leave for the day. Then tomorrow we can move onto requirements."

"Yes. I agree with Esther."

As did I.

"Sounds good to me. So here is the deal. It appears coffee and tea will be ready in five minutes. We will take a break and continue in fifteen. Deal?"

"Yes!"

I used this time to make a quick phone call, "Hi, Honey."

"Hi, Dear. How is your day going?"

"Remember the stories I shared with you from one of our members? Well, there were many more very similar in nature."

"Oh, Tom."

"Doc, we have much work to do. There are so many ways we are not only not honoring our mission but actually harming those we serve (and quite frankly we may also be harming the very people we have brought here to help others)."

"Listen to me. You sound wiped out. Just finish your work today, and then I want you to go back to your office, organize everything like you always do for the next day, but this time do not bring anything home with you. Before you leave there tonight, you just get everything ready for another day. Tomorrow is that other day. Tonight," she trailed off for a moment, "You just come home to me. I am worried about you." And then with more vigor, "Tonight there will not be any stress. You just come home to me and the kids and Angus. We will be waiting with lots of hugs and kisses."

And, of course, this got me laughing.

"Yes, Dear," I chuckled. "Whatever you say."

"I am being serious."

The aroma of coffee wafted throughout the front of the building. Clearly, the team had indulged in one of my favorite passions.

"Tom, where is your coffee?"

"I am on it, Frank. I am on it. Be back in a flash."

Over the next couple of hours, we shared and heard many more voices. Powerful, impactful, some positive, others not.

Two that standout include the first shared by Stephen:

> "I had an appointment at a practice owned by the hospital a few weeks ago…"

As a reminder, some voices we collected were from patients of other systems.

> "… and as I sat, I watched other patients who had arrived after me get seen before I was. Eventually I asked what was going on and I was told, 'we have to take care of our own patients first,' I didn't even know what that meant but clearly they did not think I was one of their patients, even though I had been seeing my doctor there for ten years."

Stephen looked up from his notes and asked the team, "What do you think they meant by 'take care of our own?'"

To which Frank replied, "I believe they are part of a system with their own self-funded health plan. And with it self-funded, financially it would be advantageous to ensure that their own member-patients are seen and kept well over any others. Perhaps that is what they meant?"

The last patient voice we heard this day was shared by Michelle, and it was from another member and patient that she and I teamed up to visit, this time with me taking the notes.

> "One and a half years ago I brought my wife," who was elderly, like her husband, "to the clinic for x-rays. While I waited in the waiting room (which, by the way, is the perfect name for it) an x-ray tech called my wife to follow her into the room for the x-ray. My wife walking with her cane followed behind her. Long story short, after her x-ray was completed the technician did not help my wife off of the table and left her alone. My wife ended up falling and breaking her hip." He had paused at this point collecting his thoughts and then continued, "Why? Tell me why someone would not help another, never mind an older woman with a cane, off of the x-ray table? Can you? Can you tell me why? Please."

"My God. I had heard about this but did not know the details. Unbelievable." And then after pausing for a brief moment, Esther continued, "Actually, and unfortunately, not unbelievable anymore." And then after one more pause, "But I am glad we know now."

We continued over another hour to process all we heard. To belay one another as we did and to use these voices as fuel in which we would improve the system.

And before we left for the day, we grouped not only these last powerful stories, but all of the voices we had processed under what we agreed was one of the most poignant and perceptive voices we had heard to date. And it happened to come from one of our oldest and most loyal military retirees:

> "I feel that I am not always valued as a customer and as a patient … but most importantly not as a person."

And we thought about that for a great while.

"We are not valuing those we should be honored to serve as a customer, as a patient, and as a person?" We repeated to one another.

"Could it be?" We said as we reviewed the culmination of our work to this point.

"Could it really be true?" We asked one another as I ensured each voice under each theme was still visible and we re-read (re-listened to) each voice we had gathered.

"This is not about a benefit," Michelle said out loud again acknowledging the painfully obvious.

"No. No, it is not. This is about much much more. This is about not valuing," Cathy paused as she took a breath, "people."

"We have created a system which does much good for sure. And we have some stories to that affect. And yet," and here I had to compose myself as I struggled a bit to finish my thought, "…and yet, we have created a system where an older woman is yelled at for requesting a coated tablet for her husband," I say as I point to the post it note where we had documented Linda Jones' voice.

"We have created a system where an elderly woman's safety is not top of mind," I say as I point to that voice.

"We created a system where those we care about are afraid or at least hesitant to ask for what they truly need."

"And we have created a system where people feel that we do not care whether they live or die."

"We have; haven't we?" Cheryl responded as I continued to follow our Language Process diagram on the wall.

"We have created a system where caring is not at the forefront of what we do and we are harming those very people we have been entrusted to care for and about and perhaps the very people we have brought together to provide the care … our doctors and nurses."

As I said this, I remember feeling my heart pounding through my chest and my face becoming flush.

Breathe, Tom. Breathe, I reminded myself as I looked around the room and continued, "And we are going to fix it."

I paused once again …

"Thank you, Team. This is a challenging project. We are going to places and learning things I don't think any of us expected. We are peaking behind a curtain that we didn't even know existed. And with the voices of our patients, we are seeing that we have much to do to bring caring back into healthcare."

As I walked around the conference room peering at what appeared to be hundreds of post-it notes, each voice visible, and yet sorted and grouped, I also looked around the room and made note that even though we were all terribly tired, there was concern but no more dismay. As I looked into the eyes of the nurse, the marketer, the developer, the finance person, and the rest of the team, I saw … resolve. And I was both proud and touched.

"We can make this right."

"Yes, Esther. We can. And we will."

"Thank you, Tom, for allowing me to be part of this process. This is the important stuff. This is why I went into healthcare. To care. And that is what we are doing."

"Thank you, Tracie."

"Ditto," Stephen then added, as the others also shared similar sentiments.

"Tomorrow we are scheduled to continue this process. This time focusing on converting these powerful voices into requirements. Those requirements that our patients and members need to ensure we are truly caring about them."

"Yes! We are moving to solution planning!" Frank excitedly responded as he punched high into the air.

"We are getting there, Frank. We are getting there," I replied in order to manage expectations as we still have much more work to do.

"Now that said, we have been going pretty hard and I know you are all carrying a full work load outside of this process. Question for you all, do you need a day to collect yourselves from this profound experience and ensure your other important work is under control?"

"Absolutely not. This is why we are here!"

REFLECTION

The data are clear, physicians and nurses are burning out, many are leaving the profession at a time when we already have a shortage of primary care physicians, nurses, and others.

And we are also losing many caring, passionate physicians to suicide.

(Estimated 1 physician suicide each and every day – Source: Medscape, Physician Suicide, Louise B Andrew, MD, JD; Chief Editor: Barry E Brenner, MD, PhD, FACEP, July 2016)

We have created a model that harms those very people we entrust to care for those we serve and those we love.

We have even harmed animal therapy dogs who were part of a VA study on the impact of this treatment approach on military personnel diagnosed with PTSD, leading to the discontinuance of the study and thus the discontinuance of some soldiers having access to beneficial animal therapy services.

Yes, the healthcare system does great good. And yet ... it is also profoundly broken. And many of us have contributed to this brokenness. And, in turn, we have created a system that does great harm.

Technical fixes such as a new financial model, quality-based incentives, additional access to health insurance, and others may serve some good.

And yet without an authentic HEARTchange of leadership throughout the health and healthcare system and beyond, and without each of our voices, we will not truly shift the paradigm in which we are currently stuck.

Questions

1. As a healthcare leader, clinician, or staff person, how do you measure "teamness?"
   a. What role have you played in enhancing a well-functioning passionate team?
   b. What would you do differently?
2. As a clinician, how have you been best positioned to care for another?
   a. In what ways has the system done you harm?
   b. How can the system better position you to care for another?
   c. Have you ever felt abused by the system?
   d. How has this abuse manifested?
3. What supports have been available to you to stop the abuse? Support you in your own healing?
4. Have you ever felt burnt out by the system? Please share a story about how you are feeling.
5. What recommendations would you make to ensure all stakeholders throughout the system are best positioned to honor their calling and care for one another?
6. As a patient or family member, when have you not felt cared for within the healthcare system? Please share a story of how this lack of caring manifested in your health and healthcare.
   a. How would you like to see the healthcare system change to improve how care is provided to you and your family?
7. As a healthcare leader, how have you maintained your integrity and ensured that your compass always pointed to what was best for all those you serve?
   a. How would you suggest other leaders follow suit?

Chapter 14

Finding the Pathway to Honor our Patients

"What a gorgeous morning. The sun is shining; the birds are chirping ..."

"And our team is back together again to make something special happen."

What a way to start the day after such a powerful, challenging, and inspirational session yesterday, I thought, as I heard Cathy share with such positivity and Esther chime right in.

"Now this is what I love to hear. Frank, what do you have for us?"

"Well, let's see, I cried more yesterday than I have ever done at work before, and I want to thank you all for that."

"Awww, Frank. Thank you for saying that. I didn't want to be the only one who felt that way," Cheryl responded as she put her arm around Frank's shoulder. Which was pretty interesting to see as Frank is probably 6' 3", and I would guess Cheryl is just a bit over 5' 2". But wonderful just the same.

"Tracie, and how are you today?"

"I am an old war horse one might say. I have been a nurse for almost thirty years and I have seen it all," Tracie began to respond, and then after a dramatic pause (*I clearly need to learn that from her as it was carried out so effectively*), she continued having looked each of us in the eyes, "but what I heard from our patient voices and combining that with how we as a team processed these nuggets of wisdom with empathy and compassion ..."

"And heart," I chimed, in not being able to hold myself back.

"Yes, and with heart, was one of the most inspiring and powerful experiences I have ever had as a nurse and as a professional."

"Yes," added Stephen and then as he chuckled, "except the 'as a nurse' part, yes, yesterday was both inspiring and powerful, and I would add, hard. Hard to learn the harm we have caused our patients, their families, and perhaps our teammates in the clinic. Hard to hear people in pain more so from our mistakes or broken processes than even from their own health challenges in many cases. Yes, very hard. But still inspirational because as a team we are going to fix this."

And then we continued our morning 'check-in' to ensure we were all whole, to ensure we were all feeling supported, to ensure we were ready to move forward, and (*don't tell anyone in business I said this*), to ensure we were all feeling both cared for and loved. Yes, loved.

"Are we ready to begin the next phase of our journey and transform our patient and member voices into prioritized requirements?"

"Once I have my coffee, I am all in!" was Stephen's response.

"Perfect. Let's get our coffee, tea, hot chocolate, or other beverage of choice and then let's get started."

And then turning to Stephen, "Love the way you think!" I said with a chuckle.

After we had each selected our favorite beverage, and some of us also a delicious pastry or two (yes, I was one of those enjoying a sweet treat …), we sat back down together and reviewed our work from the prior evening.

> Note: always keep your team well fed … or in other words … show your team you care about them in many different ways.

"Debbie, would you please walk us through our groupings from yesterday?"

The process of transforming voices into requirements is challenging at best and, after another five hours, we were all getting very tired.

Esther, "Cathy, previously you said, 'I never would have thought we were not meeting these basic requirements.' I thought that, too. But clearly those we care most about are telling us differently."

Frank interjected, "Now, not all of these requirements are saying that we currently do not completely meet the needs, but rather some are a reminder that we can do better in certain areas." Frank paused and then, "While with others, it is clear we have totally missed the boat."

Tracie added, "I am tired. And truly, we need another break. But before we do, I simply want to say that if it were not for this team and this process, we would not be aware of these opportunities." She paused that really cool, dramatic pause I like and then said, "So this is a good thing. Hard to see? Yes. Hard to hear? Yes. Hard to say? Yes. But necessary data in which we will make a difference. Yes. This is a very good thing."

And later after another break and another couple of hours, we arrived at the following overall Aim (requirement) to both represent and honor our patient and member voices as well as key drivers to address to ensure we achieve it.

Aim statement:

> "To have a committed and caring healthcare team caring about me as a whole person and providing me with confidence in the service and care I receive."

"Team, what do you think?"

"I am personally blown away. Through this process, we have identified specific areas in which we will prioritize, develop S.M.A.R.T. goals, identify root causes, and eliminate barriers to achieving, will implement PDSAs and measure, and over time will continuously improve. And, we did it with a 'market-in' approach. We did it by truly listening to our patients and members. We have our True North. We have our Aim."

Clearly the CQM training and this process was resonating. *Fantastic!* I thought to myself.

"Thank you, Michelle."

"You have trained me well."

"Tom, we have created a pathway to innovating healthcare. And, as Michelle shared and we all know, we did it not by listening just to ourselves and to the other healthcare 'experts,' we did it by truly hearing the voices of our patients and members and marrying that with our own wisdom."

"Yes, Tracie, yes, by this team coming together, caring about one another and never losing focus on our mission, we have arrived in this special place," Debbie added.

Each member of the team shared their thoughts about the process to date and our current state, and even though mentally exhausted, each was excited to begin the next phase of this process.

"Thank you, all. And now as a reminder relative to our schedule, you each have a few days respite from this challenging and rewarding work while Esther and I head to Seattle for the military healthcare meetings …"

"Wait, what? I don't want to go back to my day job. This work is far more important and fun," Frank said with a combination of intense seriousness and a bit of jest.

"Me, either!" Cheryl and Michelle then each said in unison.

"Let me finish. Let me finish," I said with a smile as I looked into the eyes of each of my teammates. "Once Esther and I are back from Seattle, we will all come back together to carry forward this most important work. Don't worry. There is nothing else I want to do more than complete our mission together."

"That's right, Tom. Agreed."

"Thank you, Esther. During the time we are away, please rejuvenate. Focus on your own health. I know you have each been essentially working two full-time jobs. And then let's come back together healthy and refreshed and change the world." This time I intentionally inserted a pause as I scanned the room before continuing, "Sound like a plan?"

REFLECTION

Similar to my team's understanding that both the themes AND the individual voices are critically important to understand and to honor when improving care, patient experience, growth, etc., it is just as critical that we do not lose the individual patient as healthcare moves more and more toward a 'system' focus and population health. 'Cookie cutter' clinical algorithms and protocols in the guise of following evidenced-based medicine based on clinical research output of an "average patient" places many in harm's way as there is NO true average patient. We are all complex adaptive beings with thousands of differing internal and external forces and influences impacting our lives.

Thus, the need for a fluid system, which balances the great macro wisdom with the additional wisdom and knowledge of the individual patient leading to a co-developed care plan specific to meeting the patient's goal(s).

We must not lose sight of the individual as the focus turns to population health.

To paraphrase Star Trek: "The needs of the many should not outweigh the needs of the one."

Questions

1. As a healthcare leader, clinician, or staff person, how often have you found yourself part of a team where you felt whole, safe, and positioned to make a difference?

    a. What were the keys to creating this environment?

2. As a healthcare leader, clinician, or staff person, how have you ensured the individual patient and family has not been lost as the system has moved toward a population health focus?

    a. Why is this (or is this not) important to you?

3. As a healthcare leader, clinician, or staff person, when have you found joy at work?

    a. What were the keys elements that manifested the joy?

    b. How important is joy in your work to you?

4. As a healthcare leader, or clinician, how do you keep your team motivated?

    a. Do you believe it is possible to motivate a team, or is motivation an internal process?

Chapter 15

The Flight

"Are you ready for this? This is your first time; isn't it," she joked.

"How are you so chipper this time of the morning, Esther?"

We were at the Portland International Jetport. It was just after 5:00am and Esther, our liaison with the Department of Defense, was a pro at this and was updating me on the trip before us.

With a big smile and laugh, "We will be traveling through Philly and then cross country to Seattle for the meetings. We will be meeting with each of our sister organizations. Our attorney from your old law firm will be present. And each day we will be focusing on improving the program and our position with the DoD."

And for the next 45 minutes (both pre-flight and while on the plane) Esther, the old (in length of service only) Contract Administrator, reviewed with me, the fairly new COO of this program (having been in the role for the last seven months) all of the goals, strategies, plans, and tactics we co-developed with our team for these meetings.

"Thank you, Esther. All of our pre-work, all of your relationship building, planning, and contract management, and all of our team's preparation has positioned us well."

"That's my job."

Prior to leaving home that morning, Doc had again noted how tired I looked.

"I am fine. Just didn't sleep well last night. And I have a little heartburn. I may have overindulged with the coffee and pastry during yesterday's marathon meetings."

"But you have been tired for quite a while. And what about the additional stressors you shared?"

"Additional stressors?"

"The organizational push to implement and leverage new technology and move to shorter office visits for all patients. I know how that has bothered you. I see how this direction is causing you stress. I see all the work you are doing to prevent this decision from becoming a reality with your team. I am a nurse you know."

"We cannot sacrifice patient safety for technology and additional revenue generation. It is against our mission. It is against our values. It is completely contrary to what our patients both want and need …"

"Honey," Doc then said very quietly. "Please. You'll figure it out. But for now, you need to relax. You need to sleep. Be sure to sleep on the plane. You need to rest."

"I will. I promise."

"Then go kick ass in Seattle, and when you are done come home to me."

"Esther, I am going to close my eyes for a bit."

Doctor's orders. Or at least my Doc's orders, I joked with myself.

"Okay, Tom. See you in Philly."

And for the rest of the first leg of our trip, I slept.

"Hagler comes out for the third Round."

"Who is he fighting?" I ask nobody.

"They are in the center of the ring. Hagler throws a right and then a left which catches Tommy squarely in the nose."

"Tommy? Tommy who?"

"It's broken. It's broken. Hagler broke Tommy's nose!"

"But this isn't Tommy 'Hitman' Hearns. This is …"

"Now body shots. A right. A left. A right. Tommy is defenseless. The body. The body. The body. I don't know what is keeping him up!"

"We will be arriving at gate B13. That is concourse B, Gate 13."

God, I can barely breathe. I must be getting sick. Doc was right, as always, I remember thinking after waking to the pilot's announcement.

"How are you doing, Esther? Did you sleep?"

"I am doing fine. Been reading over the latest contract documents."

She was so good. Esther was perfect for the Contract Administrator role. Her background, knowledge, passion, ability to connect, and so much more ... perfect.

"How are you?"

"I am fine. It was good to shut my eyes for a bit. I see our layover is Philly is over an hour long. Want to get breakfast?"

"Absolutely."

My kind of travel companion.

"Tom, you are looking a little pale. Are you okay?"

"Yes. Just a bit tired and hungry and, my god, is it hot in here!"

"Actually, it is not, Tom."

And then when it was our turn to proceed up the aisle, "You go ahead, Esther. It's going to take me a few minutes. You know, the old football injuries and all."

The first time having an old injury ever came in handy.

"Okay. I will be just inside the concourse scoping out our breakfast joint."

I really must be getting sick, I remember thinking to myself as I grabbed the empty seat in front of me and pulled myself up. *My back hurts. My knees hurt. My shoulder ... come to think of it all my joints hurt. And this pressure on my chest, I can barely breathe. Time for some ibuprofen with breakfast. Hope I can take it with my Vioxx and keep them both down."*

"Are you okay, sir?"

"Oh, yes. Joints are just a bit stiff this morning."

"Okay. Please move along then. We need to get this plane cleaned for our next flight."

"Understood. I just need to get my bag from the overhead, and I am good to go."

But unfortunately, my back was really cramping at this point, and I was having trouble breathing.

"Let me get that for you, sir."

And then with one bag over my shoulder and the other being pulled from behind, I made my way off of the plane … very slowly.

So far so good, I remember telling myself as I entered the jet way. But then I quickly realized that the slight upward slope toward the entrance to the terminal was going to be a problem.

I just need to rest here and catch my breath for a minute, I said out loud to nobody in particular as I began to become lightheaded.

Damn, I must really have the flu.

"Tom, you made it. What took you so long?"

"Sorry about that, Esther. Did you find a place for breakfast?"

"Sure did. And it is really close to our gate."

"That is great, Esther. I really want some waffles."

"Well, Tom, that is the bad news. They don't serve waffles."

Together Esther and I sat for the next thirty minutes. We enjoyed coffee and our non-waffle-based breakfast as we continued our discussion about the week ahead.

"I am very much looking forward to seeing the different approaches each of our sister organizations are using to engage their members. How they are retaining them and how they are increasing access for new members," I said.

"You should have plenty of opportunity to learn much. Each site being different will lead to different approaches."

"True, Esther, but the core value proposition should shine through. And I am eager to see how each is living its values as it seeks to achieve its mission. Many say, 'no margin, no mission'. Let's see if any also embrace 'no mission, no margin.'"

We continued this discussion as I struggled to hide between sentences just how difficult I was finding it to breathe.

"We better get to our gate. We don't want to be late."

"Are you okay, Tom?"

"Actually, I think I am coming down with something. Let me just catch my breath. And I would recommend you don't sit next to me on the next leg of our trip."

"Don't worry about me. Let's get you feeling better. We need you healthy for the meetings. How about some tea?"

Within fifteen minutes I had finished my tea, and we had made it onto our next flight. And aside from embarrassing myself by not being able to put my bag in the overhead compartment, all was good.

"You okay now, Tom?" Esther asked as she settled in diagonally behind me.

"Oh yes. The tea was very helpful, and with a few more hours of sleep, I should be ready to go," was my response as I tried to convince both Esther and myself that I would feel better shortly.

"The captain has turned off the fasten your seatbelt sign …"

Oh good. I can stretch out a bit more now, I thought as I listened to the flight attendant. I was tired, I was in pain, and sweat was dripping down my forehead. And beyond that, a pressure on my chest was worsening as I struggled to breathe.

"Sir, would you like a beverage?"

"Yes. A water would be great. Could I also get a couple of pillows and a blanket?"

"Absolutely. I will be right back."

I figured if I could just get comfortable, I would be able to sleep and then feel better upon awakening.

"Here you go, sir. Here are your pillows and your blanket. And here is your water."

I took the water and placed it on my tray table. I then rolled the blanket up and place it in the curve of my lower back. And then I positioned the first pillow (the one I already had) behind my right trapezoid, the second pillow behind my surgically repaired left shoulder, and the third pillow I leaned my head against as I tried to find an equilibrium and peace.

This will provide comfort for a while, I told myself as I also continued to listen to my mother's words from so long ago, *Keep breathing, Tom. Keep breathing.*

But no matter what I did, I just couldn't seem to get comfortable.

So instead I pulled out the ample paperwork for this week's meetings and tried to concentrate on the contract language, negotiation positions, business models, fee schedule analyses, network adequacy stats, and member satisfaction data.

"Ma'am, I am sorry to be a pain but could I have some ice for my water?"

"Are you not feeling well?"

"I think I may be coming down with something."

Surely not what the flight attendant wanted to hear, but she was very kind and proceeded to get me another cup of water along with a cup of ice.

"Here you go, sir. Just relax and let me know if you need anything. We have just over another four hours until we reach our destination. There will be a food service in another couple of hours, but you let me know if you need anything in the meantime."

Wow. Airline passenger-centered care? I thought to myself. *Perhaps a new tagline for the airline, 'We provide passenger-centered care each and every flight for each and every passenger.'*

And then an entire process and system in which to ensure it evolved came to mind. I could picture it ... *Prior to each flight we leverage technology to get to know each our customers. We then leverage this information as our team of flight attendants focus on developing an authentic connection with each of our customers to ensure passenger preferences and needs are known and honored.*

Just as Mary, my flight attendant, did with me.

Thank you, Mary. I said to myself as I again tried to close my eyes but this time feeling a bit better knowing someone was looking out for me.

As the flight continued and after numerous yoga type maneuvers to get my back, chest, and shoulder settled and to ease my breathing, I decided I needed to get up to use the restroom.

But as I tried to get up, I realized this time the exertion was just too much for me.

Are you kidding me? I thought as my chest felt like it would explode and I gasped for air. *Get up!* I yelled in my head as I used both of my arms, my legs, the back of the seat in front of me ("Sorry for disturbing you, sir"), and the two empty seats in my row to push and pull and claw my way into a standing position.

"Can I help you?"

I must have looked pathetic.

"I simply need to get to the restroom."

"Are you okay?"

"I really don't feel very good."

I was so glad Esther appeared to be sleeping and thus not witnessing this.

"Let me help you."

Passenger-centered care at its finest.

"I am okay. I just need to catch my breath."

"Okay. My name is Mary." I had already read Mary's nametag, but her sharing her name with me meant a great deal. "Please let me know if I can help."

"I will. I just need a moment. Thank you."

And as Mary turned to assist another passenger …

Okay. It looks like maybe 20 steps. I can do this, I told myself.

One. Two. Okay. Rest.

Three. Four. Okay. Another Rest. God, I must look pathetic.

Five. Six. I am now past Esther. She didn't say anything. I think she is sleeping. Okay. Good.

And I repeated this process over and over until I got to the restroom.

Vacant. Thank God, I said to myself.

Now I don't know if you ever noticed, but the restroom doors on an airplane are actually quite heavy.

Damn.

But with a little elbow grease (at least I believe that is the term) I was able to push and pull the door open and squeeze myself into the linen closet space I remembered as a child that is now referred to as a restroom.

Okay. I made it. Now I will just lean on the wall for a bit until I can catch my breath. Hopefully no one is waiting.

And then very hesitantly I looked into the mirror.

I looked awful. Almost grey. And wet. And much older than I looked 24 hours ago. Or at least I thought.

Don't pee on yourself! I demanded as both of my legs shook. *That is all you need. I can see it now, 'Who is that guy that smells like sweat and urine? And why can't he walk straight?'*

On the way back I repeated the same process but in reverse until I reached my row and collapsed across my three seats once again.

Made it!

A few hours later I was awoken by, "Please place your seat trays in their upright and locked positions …"

I slept. Thank God, I slept.

"Sir, you missed the food service. Would you like some pretzels? Can I get you anything?"

"I am okay. But thank you, Mary."

"Okay. Please make sure your seat back is in its full upright position. And make sure your seatbelt is fastened. We don't want you getting hurt."

The plane continued its descent with only slight shimmying and shaking and within 15 minutes we were taxiing toward the terminal.

"Tom," I wondered how Mary knew my name, "Here is another water for you. Take care of yourself here in Seattle. Your family will want you to come back to them safe and sound."

Yes, passenger-centered care.

REFLECTION

I believe it was at the Center for Quality Management (CQM) in Cambridge when I first heard the saying about begging and borrowing (appropriately) good ideas to make things better.

And it was truly fascinating, as well as dichotomous, to first witness Saul bringing manufacturing concepts into healthcare with the idea to "borrow" these quality improvement ideas and processes (that we were paying handsomely for via CQM) and use them to improve the care for our patients, while also seeing (and continuing to see) so many healthcare systems literally, as per many doctors, patients, and others I have interviewed over these last fifteen years, turn doctors into production workers, patients into widgets, and healthcare systems into factories.

Truly, when one appropriately borrows ideas from other industries for the benefit of others, it is both wise and of service (servant leadership) due to the True North of mission and congruency of intention and action.

And now, reflecting back to the flight attendant and the "passenger-centered care," I again see how person-centered care transcends industries and, when done well, positively impacts both the giver and the receiver.

Questions

1. As a healthcare leader, clinician, or staff person, what congruencies do you see between the airline industry and the healthcare system?

    a. What lessons can the airline industry learn from the healthcare system?

    b. What lessons can the healthcare system learn from the airline industry?

2. As a patient or family member, is it important to you to feel that your doctor or nurse truly cares about you?

    a. Is it important to you that the clinicians working within your healthcare system care about their patients and families?

    b. Is it important to you that your care team cares about one another? Why or why not?

    c. Would the "caring" still be authentic if they were being paid specifically to do so?

    d. In what industries beyond healthcare is it also important to you to feel cared for?

Chapter 16

Military Maneuvers

"Tom. I will meet you in the jet way."

"Esther," I wanted to say but could not as my chest gripped tight. So, I just nodded.

Even with the kindness of Mary and my nap, this leg of our travels had taken a lot out of me, and I was unsure if I could walk off this plane on my own.

This thought terrified me.

"Sir?"

"Please go ahead," I responded to the gentlemen sitting behind me as he offered to let me disembark ahead of him.

The pressure on my chest was growing stronger now as was the pain in my back.

Relax. Keep breathing. Don't stress. Deep breaths. Take slow deep breaths. Once everyone clears, you can take your time and get up and leave, I coached myself.

"Tom, can I help you?"

"Mary, I am really not feeling well. I just need a little extra time if that is okay."

"Where is your overhead bag? I will get it for you."

"Right above me. Thank you."

"Tell you what, I will carry it to the door. You just take your time. Okay?"

I waited for Mary to get out of earshot, as I knew it would take all I had to just stand up and pull myself to the aisle, and grunting like I was back in the gym in doing so would not be the ideal.

Slowly, actually very slowly, I made it up the aisle and to Mary at the doorway.

"Here is your bag, Tom. Thank you for flying with us. And be sure to take good care of yourself."

"Tom! I didn't see you behind me, so I came back. Are you okay? You look awful."

"I think I might have the flu. I am hurting all over and can't catch my breath."

"Well, let's get you to the hotel as quickly as possible so you can lay down. You'll feel better after a good night's sleep."

Of course, it was only midafternoon West Coast Time, but Esther's plan sure did sound good.

"Esther, I don't want you to get sick. Why don't you go on ahead to the hotel, and I will see you in the morning at the first meeting?"

"No. We are traveling together. I am not leaving you."

What else would I expect from someone with a military background?

I continued to walk precariously slow and feel even more terrible about being a burden to Esther than I did about the pain I was in.

And after what felt like a 10-mile hike through the terminal, but in reality, was probably more like a tenth of a mile, I was beat.

"Esther, I need to stop," I gasped. "I am so sorry."

"Tom, it is okay. We got this."

"Yes, we got this. Together," is what my standard operating procedure would be. And what I would typically respond. But not at this time.

At this time an overwhelming sense of dread was coming over me like a black cape engulfing my mind, my soul and my heart. And all I want to do was get home to my wife and kids.

"Tom? Are you okay? Why are you holding your chest?!"

Cough. Cough. Cough.

"Esther, please go and hail us a cab."

"I am not leaving you."

"Please."

After drifting off in the cab, I awoke with a start.

"Esther, Let's go someplace near Pike's Place Fish Market for lunch. The place that became famous for throwing fish."

I was feeling guilty for the worrying Esther was doing about me. And I also wanted to witness firsthand their values that espoused …

"… going beyond just providing outstanding service to people. It means really being present with people and relating to them as human beings."

"Sounds great, Tom, but only if you are up to it."

Esther and I had a very nice low-key lunch (and did get to see the World Famous Fish Market) and eventually we arrived at our hotel.

"Esther, I am quite tired, so I think I will just check in and go to bed. Would you mind letting our associates who we are intending to join for dinner know that I am a bit under the weather and that I will see them in the morning."

"Of course, Tom. Get some sleep, and I will see you in the morning."

Lucky for me we were staying in the same location where all the meetings would be taking place.

"Hi, Doc."

"Hi, Honey! So great to hear from you. How are you? How were your flights?"

"Doc, I am feeling very tired. I think I am going to go to bed."

"It is still very early out there. Are you okay?"

"I might be coming down with something."

"Okay, honey. Just take care of yourself. I love you."

Once I had changed and gotten into bed, I fell asleep very quickly and slept soundly until …

"Oh my God. My chest!" I cried out loud as an intense pressure on my chest took hold.

"Doc!" I yelled like I would do when my head was going to explode from the pain in my neck and shoulder. "Doc, please help me," I cried out as the pressure became pain. "Please… "

Okay. Okay. You can do this. Just get to your phone and call 911.

"No! No! You just have the flu."

Back and forth I went. "Call!" "No. It's the flu."

Just get through the night. Just get through this night. One moment at a time. Suck it up and get through the night. The team is counting on you, I stoked myself. *Be strong. You can do this.*

Breathe Tom. Breathe. And sleep. Go back to sleep. You will feel better. Sleep.

Beep Beep Beep Beep

"What is that? Where am I?"

"It's morning. I made it. I made it through the night," I congratulated myself.

But then as I fully arrived into my body, the sledgehammer hit again.

Okay. I can do this. We have breakfast at 7:30am and then meetings from 8:00am until Noon and then from 1:00pm to 4:30pm each day.

"I will skip breakfast and go to the morning meetings. If I am not feeling better, I will come back to the room and nap until 12:45pm and then rejoin the team.

And that was the game plan I used to get through each day of these important meetings in Seattle. I woke. Grabbed something small to eat on the way into the meetings. Focused and participated as much as physically possible during the morning sessions, went back to bed at lunch, and then again participated in the afternoon sessions each day prior to going back to my room, calling my bride, and then going back to bed.

Each day. Every day.

And each night I prayed …

"Lord, Please help me get through this week. Please give me the strength."

And by the time Esther and I touched down back in Portland, I was as grey as a storm cloud (mentally and physically), clammy and shaking, and feeling as if I had gone fifteen rounds with Rocky (Marciano, of course, not Balboa). I was so ready to be home.

"Oh my God, Tom. You look awful."

"I'm okay."

"You are not okay. We are getting you home and into bed right now."

REFLECTION

Not too long ago I was invited to a meeting of experts to discuss how best to improve patient and family engagement in healthcare at a system level.

I remember walking into the meeting room and being pleased to see that I was slated to sit next to the meeting co-chair, who I had met previously and wanted to get to know even better.

As I walked out to stow my luggage, one of the meeting coordinators approached me and let me know that they were moving me because another individual required access to a plug (which happened to be right behind the seat I was initially assigned to).

I remember being a bit disappointed but thinking "No big deal ... I will simply connect with the co-chair later in the day."

Interesting how fate works.

Shortly thereafter, I realized I would be sitting next to a brilliant patient advocate, who also happened to have a chronic degenerative neurological disease. (I will refer to him as Neal.) And throughout the day, Neal showed all of the following symptoms of the disease:

- Tremors
- Bradykinesia
- Rigid muscles
- Impaired posture and balance
- Loss of automatic movements
- Speech challenges

As the meeting began, I became aware of Neal's breakfast. How he appeared to struggle with his fruit. How the juice cup in his hand flailed precariously close to being dumped on him, on me, and/or on the table. And I realized I had no idea how to help. I had no idea whether Neal wanted help. Would I offend him by offering help? What was Neal's preference?

As the day went on, Neal confided in me that he was getting tired, and I noted his symptoms worsening. He stood up abruptly and his chair, which was on wheels, flew backward so I grabbed it and held it for him. I saw him stumble and thought he would fall, so I reached out and held his arm. Neal brought out a pill container, and I thought he was having some difficulty extracting his pills but decided to hold off at first on offering assistance. Again, I wasn't sure what he would want and whether he was finding my persistent questioning, e.g., ...

- *"Can I help you?"*
- *"How can I assist?"*
- *"Can I get that for you?"*

... bothersome.

He retrieved his pills on his own. He then began to lean toward me, and I asked again "can I help you," but received no answer.

A bit later Neal handed me a can of soda and asked me to open it for him, which I was happy to do. And yet, as I did so I noticed he also had a cup of ice and based on what I was witnessing, I was thinking there was no way he would be able to pour the drink into his cup without spilling. And as I was about to ask him if he wanted me to do it (feeling more comfortable after a number of hours together), Neal leaned over to me and asked me to do so for him.

I remember thinking how interesting the thoughts are that go through your mind during these times.

Feeling that at any moment I could be wearing Neal's drink, I made a pact with myself that if it does happen I will not show any manifestation of being startled, I will not immediately get up and go clean my suit, but rather I will take it in stride and ensure that I do not cause any sort of scene that would adversely impact Neal. Or, in other words, I will do my best to treat Neal how I would want to be treated in lieu of not truly knowing Neal and his preferences.

At the end of a long day I noticed Neal circling me. He came near and then circled away. He came near and then stumbled (and I supported him) and then circled away again. He then stopped nearby, and we made eye contact and he simply said, "Tom, I want to shake your hand," which we did and I responded, "Neal, it was so great to meet you."

During a long commute home, I continued to process these events.

I was blessed to be sitting with my new colleague. I was fortunate to be further reminded throughout the day of how important it is to develop relationships, to develop trust, to share openly and honestly, and to understand one another's whole story, preferences, goals, desires, and so much more ... and especially so in healthcare. I learned that the more I got to know Neal and understand his preferences the better I felt and the better I was able to respond accordingly and meet his needs more effectively.

Questions

1. As a healthcare leader, when was the last time you truly engaged at the patient encounter level? What is stopping you?

2. As a clinician, when was the last time you felt you had the time and tools to truly and authentically connect with your patient? What will you do by Tuesday to address any barriers to this connection?

3. As a patient, when was the last time you truly felt listened to and a partner in the development of your care plan? When was the last time you felt that your preferences (and you) were treated with respect within the healthcare system?

4. What would you recommend to ensure all stakeholders within the healthcare system, e.g., doctors, nurses, other staff, patients, families, communities, and others are all listened to and treated with respect and dignity as they too treat others similarly.

Chapter 17

Home from Seattle

I don't recall much of the landing in Portland except for the warmth of holding my bride again.

The ride home was also a blur. I may have slept. I am not sure. All I remember is the repeated horse kicks to the chest.

"You are breathing so heavy," Doc said as we pulled into our garage.

"You take my breath away."

"Stop it. I am serious."

"Daddy! Daddy! Daddy's home! Momma! Daddy's home!" Tommy dressed in his Superman pajamas yelled as Doc helped me into the house.

"Sammy! Haylee! Daddy's home! Daddy's home!" Tommy chanted as he kangarood. "Come see Daddy!"

"Daddy!" Sammy cried out next as she ran to me in her pink princess pajamas and with her hair perfectly in place in a pink barrette.

And then Haylee. "Daddy," She called out as she casually strolled around the corner with her Lion King in her arms.

"Tommy, Sammy, Hay Hay," I missed you so much. "And yes, Angus, you too," I said as Angus jumped up and nearly knocked me off my feet as I held three of my blessings.

"Daddy! Daddy! Daddy! Pick me up! Pick me up!"

"Me too, Daddy! Me too, Daddy!" Sammy and Haylee then said in unison.

"Kids, your father isn't feeling well. He loves you but needs to go to bed ... now! Tell him you hope he feels better."

"Love you, Daddy. We missed you this much," Sammy said while spreading her arms wide.

That's my Sammy.

"Aw Mom, I want to play with Daddy!"

That's my Tommy.

"Okay, Momma. Love you, Daddy."

That's my Haylee.

And as Doc helped me to bed, she said, "Our Deacon said 'in sickness and in health'. When is the 'in health' part going to start?"

"Ahhhhh!!!"

"Tom. What's wrong, honey? What's wrong?"

"I'm okay."

"I heard you yell."

For the remainder of the weekend I stayed in bed hiding my chest pain, breathing difficulties, and dry cough.

I've got to be better for Monday. I am sure I did not perform well in Seattle, and I want to make things right with Esther and my team.

"Tom, there is no way you are going to the office today," Doc said as she saw me trying to get out of bed Monday morning.

"I will be fine."

"No. No, you won't. I hear you cough. You cannot hide it from me. You are staying in bed today. And by the way, I have already made the call and let them know you are sick and will not be in."

"But ..."

"No buts!"

And that is how the rest of the week played out as well. Each day I tried to go to work, and each day Doc played the warden.

REFLECTION

In healthcare we talk about patient AND family engagement quite a bit. "We MUST engage the patient AND the family to ensure optimal care."

And yet ...

Not all families are the same. Just as not all patients are the same. Nor doctors or nurses. Nor any one of us.

In fact, there are many families that are not healthy and not in a position to be part of a support system for our patients.

Thus, it is critically important to create a system which allows for optimal understanding of the patient and the family along with the dynamic therein.

With this understanding, and together with the patient, we can determine how best (or not) to engage the family in the care journey at present while also ensuring each member of the family also has access to services (healthcare or other) they may need, which ideally will lead to their optimal health in the long run and a healthier supportive family unit as a whole.

Questions

1. As a healthcare leader, clinician, or staff person, how important is it to understand the patient's family dynamic and support system?

    a. What approach would you recommend to learning this information?

    b. And once learned, how would you use this information to best support the patients healing processes?

Chapter 18

Back in the Office

The ride to the office was quiet except for the occasional "Isn't Simba cute?" or "What are we doing for lunch, Mommy?" from Haylee.

"Tom. Call me if you feel any worse. Maureen and I will be looking at those houses I showed you last night, but I will come and get you whenever you need. Understand?"

"Of course, Doc. But it has been a week. I will be fine."

"Hey, Tom!"

"Good morning, Lisa."

"We have missed you. I heard the meetings in Seattle went very well. Congratulations."

They did?

"I also heard you have not been feeling well." And then almost in a whisper, "And honestly, you still look under the weather."

"I am much better. Thank you."

"Tom! I have missed you. Are you feeling better?"

"Good morning, Esther. Yes. Much better. Thank you."

"You looked awful out in Seattle," Esther said as I see her scanning my face through her glasses. "Are you sure you are feeling better? You are still looking quite grey."

"I am on the mend," I replied as I felt another Hagler jab to my chest.

"Well. Okay, but I also wanted to let you know that we received very positive feedback from our trip."

"That is wonderful, Esther." I responded as I was thinking, *God, I wish I could remember. I wish I could recall how brilliant, I am sure, Esther was. I wish I could share specifics of her impact on us having a successful meeting.* But for the life of me I couldn't.

"Esther, thank you for all of your preparations. All of your hard work. For all you did to position us for success. I am so very grateful."

The next thing I knew I was sitting in a chair, sweating and trembling in the cubicle of my good friend Tory Vard, our Manager of Medical Services.

Until Mandy Blake, one of our medical management nurses, stopped by, took one look at me …

"Tom. You are getting in my car right now."

"But …"

"Listen to me. You are getting in my car. I am taking you to the emergency room right now!"

REFLECTION

"My doctor says I'm non-compliant," she sobbed.

This 40-year-old woman had recently been diagnosed as morbidly obese and told she was at risk for heart disease and diabetes. "If I don't change my ways, I know I won't be around to see my children grow up. But now my doctor told me I'm 'non-compliant' because I don't eat according to the diet she prescribed or get enough exercise. I am so ashamed; I don't know what to do."

In the mid-to-late 2000's, as the executive director of a small nonprofit research organization and innovation laboratory, I saw patients share this scenario with our clinicians quite often. Patients felt desperate, shamed, and alone. The exact opposite of what they should expect and require of our health care system: the exact opposite of a healthCARING model.

So it was no surprise to me when, as part of the NPR series, What Shapes Health?, I read the story "Can Family Secrets Make You Sick?" and made note of the impact of Adverse Childhood Experiences, or ACE, on adult health. In too many cases, women and men who are considered "non-compliant" by the traditional medical system were victims of abuse as children. For example, experiencing sexual abuse as a child can lead a person to have an insecure relationship with her or his body and thus with food (such as the 40-year-old woman noted above). Those who have been bullied by coaches and others during youth sports may end up with severe distaste for exercise. But physicians rarely hear about these experiences, and thus do not understand these barriers in their patients' way.

And why don't physicians hear about these experiences? One key reason is that we have not created health care systems that allow for adequate time with each patient. In order to recoup the cost of doing business, many physicians see anywhere between 30 and 60 patients per day. Many primary care physicians are actually triple-booked every fifteen minutes to ensure that these productivity measures are met.

This healthcare model simply does not allow enough time for a doctor and patient to create a relationship. And without this relationship, trust is not developed.

Without time, relationship and trust, patients do not feel safe enough to tell their whole story.

And without the whole story, in this example, physicians do not understand why their patient is obese and why their patient is not modifying their nutrition plan or sticking to their exercise program.

Instead, these patients are often labelled as non-compliant which, in some cases, leads to being discharged from the practice, even though the patient was both engaged and activated (to use two current healthcare industry buzzwords).

We can do better- and many are trying every day. The Patient Centered Medical Home (PCMH) is an example of an innovation with the intention to evolve this model. The IHI Triple Aim of improving experience, quality, and cost of care is also a step forward, since it focuses as equally on patient experience as it does on population health and per capita costs (which, of course, are all connected).

> *[NOTE: An important improvement to the Triple Aim would be the focus on the health and well-being of doctors and nurses and other healthcare workers, as well as refocusing the often misunderstood and misapplied concept of patient experience with a true healthCARING model]*

In 2010, I spoke with other healthcare leaders about these stories of patients' childhood abuse and the impact on their health; the label of non-compliant we thrust upon them; and their resulting feelings of abandonment, self-loathing, and shame. I also had the opportunity to share the term "relationship-centered care" at that time, and the importance of ensuring that we build into any new care model the space for time, relationship, continuity, trust, empathy, safety and compassion.

We discussed the importance of each of these components and how together, they allow:

- *for whole stories to be told and heard;*
- *for clinicians to reconnect with their own passion for healing;*
- *for the socioeconomic and environmental factors impacting optimal health and healing to be identified;*
- *for issues such as abuse to be raised and discussed;*
- *and for the clinician and patient (and family) to co-create a care pathway that addresses the root cause of the health challenges and is aligned with patient preferences.*

And how in doing so, we position the patient for adherence, engagement, activation and most importantly, optimal health.

While this message was not ready to be heard in 2010, I was delighted to receive an e-mail recently from a national healthcare leader with a link to the research article "Relationship-centered care: A new paradigm for population health management" and to read the authors' conclusion:

"As we move toward value-based care, the combination of relationship-centered care and patient-centered care should be considered foundational to healthcare delivery innovation, especially when these kinds of innovations are closely tied to population health management."

It is not too late for this model to be created, and together we can make it happen.

Questions

1. As a healthcare leader, what systems have you created to ensure clinicians and patients are best positioned for optimal connection and maximum adherence to care protocols? Is it successful? How do you know?

2. As a clinician, what will you do today to ensure that "non-compliant" patient's whole story is listened to and understood? How will you then best use this additional information to partner with your patient to co-create a new care pathway for maximum adherence?

3. As a patient or family member, what do you see your role is in ensuring you are best positioned to achieve your health goal? What will you do to maximize your potential in doing so?

Chapter 19

The Healthcare Alphabet

"Doc, they said they are ruling out a heart attack."

"A heart attack? Oh, Tom …"

The fog was lifting more and more as my cell transmogrified back into an emergency room bay, and I looked into those beautiful eyes that had captured my heart eleven years ago. They were filled with tears now but still that beautiful ice blue.

"I'm okay. I just have the flu. I'm okay," I assured as I reached out my punctured left arm and touched the love of my life.

"A heart attack? No. You did not have a heart attack."

"I am so sorry they called you. Soon they will rule out anything bad and then we can go home."

Of course, the code being called next door, the beeping of the heart monitor behind me, the hospital gown hanging off my frame, the visible ECG leads, the other leads still connected to the pulsing heart monitor, the large needle in my left arm attached to the clear tube feeding me ice cold fluid, the band aid in the crease of my right elbow where they recently drew blood, the blood pressure cuff on my right arm, and the pulse oximetry gadget on my right index finger didn't necessarily put either of us at ease.

Being a nurse, much of this was not new to Doc. And being a frequent flyer (as one might say), much of this was not new to me either.

But for Doc and me both hearing that I may have had a heart attack and seeing me attached to all these machines … that was new. Brand new.

"Doc, why don't you go get the kids from Maureen and go home. They'll release me soon."

Well, as soon as I said it, I knew it was ridiculous, but let's just say I was not necessarily thinking optimally.

"I am not going to leave you," came Doc's reply which of course made me think of Maverick in Top Gun, "I am not leaving my wingman." In fact, it almost made me chuckle.

"I know. I am sorry I said that. I just don't want you to worry. I will be fine."

The curtain was thrown back again with what was that familiar Star Trekkian swoosh and in stepped a tall dark-haired man in his late fifties with a white coat and silver glass frames.

"Mr. Dahltrub, I am Dr. Mewnfrys. I have read your test results. Your cardiac enzymes are elevated. We are keeping you overnight. My nurse will be back in shortly."

And then … he was gone.

"Doc, what does that mean … "cardiac enzymes are elevated"?

My wife is an amazing obstetric and gynecological nurse. Unfortunately, at this moment, not a cardiac nurse.

"I don't know specifically, Tom. I will call Darl. She will know."

My sister, Darlene, is also a nurse. And luckily for us, she is a cardiac nurse.

"Unfortunately the Mylanta we gave you has not decreased your chest pain."

We didn't even see the doctor come back in.

"Your GI workup was negative. The CBC with Diff showed inflammation and we have ordered some additional tests. My nurse will be back in to apply a nitroglycerin paste to your chest to open up your blood vessels and relieve you of some of your discomfort."

And then he was gone again. And once again I found myself looking to my wife for answers.

"CBC with Diff?"

"Complete blood count with differential. It is a more in-depth blood test showing different types of blood cells. It will let us know what is happening with inflammation or infection. They are probably ordering an ANA as well as a precaution due to your family history of rheumatoid arthritis."

"Dr. Mewnfrys asked me to apply nitro paste to your chest. This should help with your pain. You may experience a headache."

A headache? I'll take a headache over this chest pain any day.

"We are awaiting some additional test results. Dr. Mewnfrys will be back in shortly. I am working on getting you a bed up on the floor. Just press the button if you need me."

"The nitroglycerin paste is placed on your chest to open up your coronary arteries. That will relieve your chest discomfort if, in fact, your chest pain is cardiac related. The headache would be from the blood vessels opening up wide and the rush of blood to your head."

"Thank you, Doc."

Well, it didn't take long …

"Doc, my head is going to explode."

"I know. I know. I don't think they can give you anything else for it. The IV should help to a certain extent."

"The additional test results are back. Your ANA is elevated. We will be observing you overnight. Any questions?"

Any questions? I had a thousand questions … and I had no questions. My head was spinning and pounding.

But all I could say was, "No, doctor. No questions," as Doc held my hand.

"Okay. My nurse will be back in shortly after she has a bed on the cardiac floor secured for you."

And then after Dr. Mewnfrys had left, "Doc, what is an ANA?"

"ANA stands for 'antinuclear antibodies'. In most cases, a positive ANA test indicates that you are having an autoimmune reaction of some kind."

Great. Chest pain. A killer headache. And now, an autoimmune reaction.

"Tom, I just spoke to your sister, she said low levels of cardiac enzymes and proteins are normally found in a person's blood stream. When the heart muscle is injured, the enzymes and proteins leak out of the damaged heart muscle into the bloodstream causing a rise."

REFLECTION

Why: The most important letter in the healing alphabet

I was blessed to have dinner with a skillful, heart-centered physician not too long ago. And at one point in our conversation, he looked up at me and confessed, "I assume way too much."

Of course, I could not let this seemingly disjointed comment lapse and pressed for more information.

> *"We doctors, we are great with the 'what' and the 'how' of healthcare. But we are terrible with the 'why.'" He then connected the missing "why" to his habit of making assumptions.*

> *"I can tell patients all day long that they must eat right (the what) and even how to do so, but too often I don't tell them the why. And if I do, most times I don't share the specific why that will truly touch them. The why that will actually engage my patient and lead to a change in behavior," he said. "Too often I assume I know all I need to know about my patient when I truly don't have a clue."*

This caring healer then went on to recall a recent patient visit that touched him deeply and led him to his conclusion.

A new patient came to his office. This man, in his mid-50s, was dressed shabbily, unshaven, uneducated and newly diagnosed with diabetes. My friend said he assumed he knew all he needed to know about this individual based on the patient's appearance and based on the information documented in the medical record. And with 30+ patients to see this day, it was time to get in, check off all the appropriate boxes, share his knowledge, and move on to the next patient.

> *"And then while I was working my way through the patient's checkup, the patient looked up at me and said, 'Hey Doc, you are ambidextrous.'"*

Those five words "Hey Doc, you are ambidextrous" made him stop in his tracks. Suddenly he realized this patient was both articulate and, in fact, educated. As he continued to process those five words, he also processed the encounter, what he saw, what he read in the chart, all the assumptions he had made and said to himself, "No, this is not right. I actually know very little about this patient and very little about how to best help this man."

He then acknowledged that yes, he was triple booked the rest of the day and was not scheduled to spend more than a few minutes with this patient, but he was going to take as much time as it required to connect with this patient, get to know this patient and communicate with this patient to the best of his ability (and become a physician healer again … not a factory worker). He was no longer going to assume but rather ask, listen, be open, and learn.

So, my friend sat down with this man and learned that this patient was a long-distance truck driver but due to his recent diabetes diagnosis could no longer drive the long distances and was very unhappy about this change.

My friend asked his patient if he knew what insulin was and what it did. He asked him about his Hemoglobin A1C levels and whether he knew what the numbers meant. And he took the time to explain. He asked his patient to imagine insulin as the vehicle (a truck) that delivers glucose from the bloodstream into cells that need energy … and he made a real connection with his patient.

Over the course of an hour and with much sharing and learning, this patient began to understand his disease. And with further discussion he better understood the "what" and the "how" of his illness but also the "why." Why it is important to monitor blood sugar levels. Why he feels the way he does. Why insulin is important. Why long-distance trucking is a challenge. Why eating a certain way is beneficial. Why exercise is important. Why. Why. Why.

As tears welled up in my eyes on hearing of this wonderful connection, not only to his patient but also to himself and his true calling, we discussed the reason for his many assumptions, as well as the barriers to reaching the 'why'.

In addition to owning his culpability, my friend also pointed to the limited time available to clinicians with their patients to truly connect, to establish relationship and trust, or to truly hear the patient's whole story (rather than assuming).

> *"As healthcare leaders, we have an obligation to ensure we create optimal healing models. And these models must include the 'why' … the most important letter in the healing alphabet," said my friend.*

That experience taught him that not doing so can harm patients and practitioners by creating a lack of understanding, noncompliance, and less-than-optimal outcomes.

> *"It also leads to a disconnect between clinicians and themselves (their true passions and the real reason they became healers in the first place)," he said.*

Questions

1. As a clinician, what is most important to you to ensure you are best positioned to care for your patients?
    a. What barriers exist to this process?
    b. What would you recommend to fix?
    c. How often do you explain the 'why' to your patients?
2. If a nurse, how would you improve the primary care visit?
    a. What prevents you from performing at your best?
    b. What recommendations would you make to address these barriers?
    c. How often do you explain the 'why' to your patients?
3. As a patient or family member, how challenging is it for you to understand what is being communicated during a primary care appointment?
    a. What would you like to see happen to improve the communication of information?
    b. How often do you understand the 'why' of your health and healthcare?

Chapter 20

Baseball and the Birthday Party (1997)

"We haven't found a room yet. We are working on it. Please be patient."

"Honey, I will be fine. I just need to catch my breath and get rid of this headache."

"What can I do?"

"The lights are so bright. Can we turn them off in here? And can I take something now for the headache?"

If only I could get a strong cup of Dunkin Donuts coffee and a couple of Excedrin Migraine tablets.

"I will ask to the nurse when she comes back."

"And I don't think I took my Vioxx today."

> Vioxx (or Rofecoxib) is a nonsteroidal anti-inflammatory drug approved by the FDA in 1999 and marketed by Merck & Co. to treat osteoarthritis, acute pain conditions, and dysmenorrhea. By 2004, it was withdrawn from the market over safety concerns.

For years I had been taking multiple doses of ibuprofen each day (and over time I began to take Naproxen and then eventually Vioxx) to combat the joint pain stemming from my many injuries ... and especially for my shoulder.

It was July 1997 and my son Tommy's first birthday. We had planned and set up for a wonderful celebration for our boy. (Doc doing the heavy planning and me doing the heavy setting up). Both of our extended families would be joining us along with many of our friends. It was a gorgeous day for a cookout in Berkley, Massachusetts.

We had delicious foods, (with all the guests contributing by bringing their specialties) and games to be played, including a floating duck game, (a game that includes a plethora of yellow ducks floating in a pool, some with red dots on their belly, and children taking turns selecting a duck and if they select one with a red dot getting a prize.)

Doc was so very excited for this game.

The sun was shining brightly as folks arrived for the festivities.

"Hey T, what a perfect day for your birthday. I hope you are excited. We are going to have so much fun," I said as I picked up my big boy and carried him out onto the deck and down the stairs to the back yard where everyone was gathering.

"The birthday boy! Here comes the birthday boy!" My dad joyfully yelled as he took Big T from my arms and carried him off to see his Great Mémère.

"Hey, Meat!" I said as I turned and saw one of my two best friends from Brockton.

"Beef!"

"You up for some whiffle ball?"

"You know it, Beef. Been working on my slider."

"TD!!!!"

It must be Spike. My other good friend from Brockton.

"Spiiiiiiike!!! Hope you are up for the whiffle ball tourney!"

"You know it. Been working on my slider."

What is this a conspiracy? I better learn how to hit a slider quick.

"Drink up. I'm going to go help Doc."

We all ate our fair share and then after presents were opened, *boy do I wish I still had those Hot Wheel sets from when I was a kid*, it was time for whiffle ball.

Now don't tell Doc but I was wearing one of her favorite grey t-shirts. A "New York" something or other. I liked it because it fit my chest and shoulders better than my own. And with all the bench pressing Meat, Spike and I do at the gym, a little more space in these areas is very much appreciated.

The teams were as follows:

Tommy, Meat, and me against Spike, my Dad, and my brother Jon.

And with all of us (except for Tommy) being from Brockton, we all wanted to win.

Meat and Spike were pitching for their respective teams. And yes, each throwing plenty of sliders.

Our version of whiffle ball is more like "lines" than baseball. Meaning you collect base hits and score runs based on where you hit the ball. For example, a ball hit into the woods is a homerun and a fly ball over the outfielder's head but not in the woods is a triple.

After a couple of hours of intense battling, it was now the last inning of the game. Meat was still pitching. We were winning by one run, and they had two outs. One more out, and we would win. They had invisible men on second and third. (As you know, invisible men are very important.) A double would tie the game, and a triple or homerun would win it for them.

Jon was up at bat when Meat for some reason threw a "Bill Lee *eephus* pitch" rather than his slider … and Jon crushed it.

Luckily for us he hit it downward and what could have been a homerun ended up being a hard ground ball to the first base side of the field. That said, I was shaded to the third base side and unless I "knocked the ball down" we were about to lose.

"I got this!" I called over to Meat as his head whipped around and the ball went past him.

But being slower than I used to be, due to both age and the multiple knee surgeries, I quickly realized I was not going to get there in time. And being from Brockton, as you know, losing was not an option. (Clearly Apollo 13 borrowed their famous line from us).

So of course, what did I do? I dove. Yes, I dove at thirty-one years of age to stop a whiffle ball from rolling past me during a game played with family and friends at my son's first birthday party. And in slow motion (and similar to a kickball lo those many years ago) I saw the spin of the white plastic orb as it bore down on my now horizontal self. I saw the sun reflect off the shine of the ball and into my eyes. I felt the wind and sweat on my face as I literally flew (the foot and a half, if that) and then …

… and then in unison I felt the ball hit off my two hands and remain in front of me to ensure the tying run did not score and I felt the crunch of my shoulder hitting the densely packed turf of my backyard.

We are still winning! Game still on! I remember initially thinking as the reality of the 'crunch' began to set in.

"That's a single!" Meat yelled in the distance as he retrieved the ball. "Bases loaded. Two outs. We are still up a run."

My right hand slid past my chest and up to the tip of my left delt.

So far so good.

I then slid my hand over my delt and toward my neck.

Pain was beginning to register as neurons were firing across all their respective synapses.

The tips of my fingers eventually found my collar bone. But it is not where it was supposed to be. Rather than flat in front of my trap and along my shoulder line it was sticking straight up and pressing against my left ear….

MY SON TOMMY CANNOT SEE ME LIKE THIS! Especially not on his birthday!

I began to hyperventilate.

Getting up with my right hand holding my collar bone where it now stood, I made a beeline to the front of the house.

Under the stairs I sprinted. Across the driveway and around our island of mulch, flowers, and rocks I ran until I got to the other side and hit the turf again, this time face down as I held my collar bone in place.

The first to find me in this prone position was my mom. (Isn't that always the way?)

"Tommy!?!" She whispered. "What is wrong?"

Later she would tell me that she had watched me jump up with my right hand holding my shoulder and run … and knew by the look on my face that something was seriously wrong.

"Mom," I gasped. "My collarbone is out of place. I can no longer move."

By now, my bride and a few others were huddled around me as I literally laid on my face.

"Call 911, NOW!"

Mom was clearly in command.

"You'll be okay. Don't hold your breath, Tommy."

Tommy? I must be really broken, I remember thinking.

"Keep breathing, Tommy. Keep breathing." Yes, in total control she was.

"Mom, did the kids see me?" I continued to gasp. "I don't want any of the kids and especially Tommy to see me hurt on his birthday."

"No. They are all still playing out back. They don't know. Tommy did not see," she replied as she rubbed my sweaty back.

Got to love mothers.

The pain was now shooting through my shoulder into my neck and up and into my left temple.

"Tommy, the ambulance will be her shortly."

Mom continued to be in charge. The General, one might say. But in this case, saying the word 'ambulance' was not necessarily helpful as it elevated my already cognizant level of stress.

"Tom, I am right here. You will be okay," I heard Doc say toward my backside as I remained prone with my face buried in sod, my right hand still holding my collarbone in place (against my left ear), and as I struggled to manage the pain.

"Tommy. I want you to picture the pain."

It was my mom again.

Years ago, when I lay in pain after another blown knee or a broken and dislocated thumb, my mom would help me manage the pain through a visualization technique. And as I lay prone in my front yard, she was at it again.

"Mom, I cannot picture the pain. It hurts too much."

"Tommy, listen to me."

Still in charge she was.

"Picture your pain. What color is it?"

"It's black," I struggled.

"Where is it, Tommy?"

Still calling me Tommy. I am really broken.

"Where is it, Tommy?"

"From the tip of my collar bone near my ear, into my neck, up past my left ear, and into my left temple."

"Keep breathing, Tommy. Keep breathing. Do not hold your breath."

She was tough.

"Move the black mass of pain, Tommy. Move the black mass of pain. You can do it. Picture the pain and move it."

"Okay. Okay." I grunted as I pictured the pain becoming a shape like my mother had taught me in the past. From a snake of black pain extending from my collarbone to my temple slowly I visualized it becoming a sphere of blackness retreating from my temple, pulling from the tip of my collarbone and forming in the side of my neck. Intense yes. But now, I was in control.

"Tommy, I want you to focus on the color and shape of the pain. I want you to flatten the black ball of pain into a two-dimensional circle."

I noticed I was no longer holding my breath as I responded to my mom and pictured the mass of pain becoming flat.

"Mom, the black pain mass is now a flat circle and I am moving it from my neck to the top of my head."

The goal is to control the pain in its entirety and move it all the way out of your body.

"Good, Tommy. Real good. Almost there."

At this point, I could hear sirens. Sirens from the ambulance as it approached our home fast. Not the cool wheeeee-yooooooo wheeeee-yooooooo sound of ambulances in London but rather the woo-woo-woo sound of ambulances here in Massachusetts.

"Ambulance is almost here."

The ambulance arrived and two EMTs jumped out and headed over to me.

"What happened?"

"He hurt his shoulder diving for a ball. His collarbone is up. He is most comfortable laying prone."

Mom was good.

"We will need to turn him over and get him up."

"Tommy, you need to stand up. I will help you."

The thought of rolling over and trying to get up was almost unimaginable.

"We will move very slowly."

"Okay. Mom. Okay. I can do this," I said more so for me than for her.

The EMT's eventually take me from Doc and my mother and guide me into the back of the ambulance and onto a gurney.

"We need to get a blood pressure cuff on you and start an IV. Can you pull your t-shirt up over your head?"

Doc was now in the ambulance. My mom remaining at home with our children.

"He cannot pull the t-shirt over his head. He cannot move that left arm."

Doc is good, too. And clearly now she was in command.

"Ok. Ok. We will cut the t-shirt off."

And with that, the EMT pulled out his silver medical scissors and began to cut Doc's favorite jersey from me.

"Let's get the cuff on him", he then said as he grabbed and tugged my left arm.

"Hmmmm ... too snug. We will need the bigger cuff for him."

I knew all the pounding of weights at the Y with Meat and Spike would pay off. *Yup, blood pressure cuff wouldn't even fit on me.*

It is interesting where your mind goes when in pain.

"Okay. Good. Now let's get an IV in."

We were moving now.

Away from the rest of my family.

Away from my son on his first birthday. Yes. Away from my son.

"Here we go. This will pinch a little."

The EMT began to insert the needle into my left arm. I felt the pinch but no big deal. I have had plenty of needles inserted into me over the years.

And then, "Oh shit!" he cried out as pulsating waves of blood was now shooting out of my arm.

"Damn!"

The EMT was frantic.

My arm, my leg, my exposed chest, my cut t-shirt, the EMT, the wall and ceiling of the ambulance, were all getting covered with my blood.

"Wait a minute. I got this!" He yelled as the ambulance continued to bounce its way toward Morton Hospital.

Unfortunately, for both me and the EMT, after removing the hard metal needle from the catheter, the IV tubing was not prepared for insertion and thus the line to my vein was wide open. And combining this with the automatic blood pressure cuff applied on the same arm, we had created quite a mess.

But eventually, he got it under control.

"So, what really happened to your shoulder?"

"You see, I'm from Brockton …"

REFLECTION

If you have played football at any level, or perhaps if you have a fantasy football team and all of a sudden care about sports-related injuries, you are probably familiar with the term "Unhappy Triad." The unhappy triad is a severe knee injury involving the full or partial tears of the Anterior Cruciate Ligament, the Medial Collateral Ligament, and a tear of the Medial Meniscus.

Back in 1984, while playing football, I decided to do one (or two) better. In addition to tearing the two ligaments and the cartilage listed above, I also tore the Posterior Cruciate and Medial Collateral ligaments. My orthopedic surgeon at that time said, "You literally have nothing holding your knee together."

Well, there went my dream (pipe dream that is) of joining the Dallas Cowboys as a slot receiver.

Why do I tell you this? In 1984, the surgery performed on my knee was the standard of care based on the evidence at that time — "evidence-based medicine." By 1988, this same surgery was no longer the standard of care and according to my new surgeon, was now considered malpractice. Five, six, or seven knee surgeries later (I lost count), I believe we finally have it right, but the damage has been done as has the cost to the system been accumulated. Clearly, new information has debunked previous research outcomes that led to the earlier "evidence-based" care.

This all came to mind as I recently read the results from the study shared in the journal SCIENCE, *"Estimating the reproducibility of psychological science." This study, which focuses on psychology research outcomes, notes: "Scientific claims should not gain credence because of the status or authority of their originator but by the replicability of their supporting evidence. Even research of exemplary quality may have irreproducible empirical findings because of random or systematic error." It highlights that only 25 percent of the social psychology experiments and only 50 percent of cognitive psychology studies were able to be replicated, meaning that for all the others, "the originally reported findings vanished when other scientists repeated the experiments."*

Why is this important as we seek to improve the health of our patients, families, and communities?

Because similar to the intervention for the unhappy triad, which was eventually proven dangerous, mental health interventions are based on the "evidence" stemming from psychology research outcomes. And based on this study, there is "a 64 percent failure rate even among papers published in the best journals in the field," John Ioannidis, professor of health research and policy at Stanford University, between the social and cognitive psychology studies, told THE GUARDIAN. And yet, interventions that affect patients, families, and communities remain reliant on these outcomes.

As research improves, we healthcare leaders in the meantime must develop new systems to better position clinicians, patients, families, and communities to optimize the challenging research outcomes within this broken system.

At a minimum, we need to ensure the following elements of a new healthcare paradigm are in place:

- *Physicians must have easy access to clinical research experts, with all biases clear and understood–noting there is always bias.*

- *Physicians must be educated on how best to critically review, assess, and analyze the clinical research for themselves.*

- *Physicians must have the time to invest in assessing the latest research.*

- *Physicians must have the time and space to discuss the research data and resulting varied treatment options with trusted colleagues and experts.*

- *Physicians must have the opportunity to leverage the now understood clinical research and discuss a challenging patient situation and/or a "best practice" in a safe setting with trusted colleagues.*

- *Physicians and patients (and families, when appropriate) must have the time and space to develop real relationships and trust where information flows freely and where whole stories are told, heard, and understood.*

- *Physicians and patients (and families when appropriate) must have the time and space to get to the root cause of a symptom and co-create a treatment plan that is based on accessible, valid, clear, bias-understood, and trusted clinical research outcomes that is best suited for the specific patient.*

- *Outcome goals and metrics for each specific patient must be developed together by the physician and patient (and families, when appropriate), assessed regularly, and the treatment approach modified as appropriate.*
- *Physicians must be compensated appropriately for all the above.*

We do not have the luxury of waiting for the greatly improved research model. Our patients, families, and communities are being harmed now.

Questions

1. As a healthcare leader, how are you ensuring only the best and most reliable research is being leveraged to create treatment protocols within your organization?

2. As a clinician or staff person, how are you ensuring you have full understanding of all of the challenges relative to new research findings being presented to you as evidence-based care?

3. As a patient or family member, are you aware of the biases and other challenges relative to the research that goes in to creating your treatment plan?

4. What would you recommend to improve the reliability of research outcomes and their translation into treatment protocols?

Chapter 21

Transport (1997)

We do eventually arrive at Morton Hospital, and I am wheeled into the Emergency Room with Doc right by my side.

"Tom, you know you are going to be fine."

It's funny how on these occasions I truly see the beauty which resides in my bride. Her gorgeous bright blue eyes, her perfect skin (yes with a plethora of those Irish freckles), the sweet smile that brightens up any room, her distinctive laugh, and that amazing heart (the heart of a nurse).

We are eventually placed into one of the ER bays and are alone, my wife and I, for quite some time.

"How is your pain?"

"I am still managing it with my mom's magic."

"Mr. Dahlborg, I am Linda. What did you do to yourself?"

"I dove for a ball," no need to tell the nurse that it was a whiffle ball, "and landed on my shoulder."

"Was your arm outstretched or tucked underneath you?"

Hmmm ... she is good, I remember thinking as I processed the question.

"When I landed, I did so on my left shoulder with my left arm tucked underneath me."

"Did you make the catch?" Linda then inquired as she smiled at both Doc and me.

She must be from Brockton.

"No. Knocked the ball down though," I said sadly.

"So, this wasn't a football game?" Linda said with a keen note of dejection in her voice.

"A long story," Doc chimed in.

"Well, football or not, we will need to x-ray that shoulder and arm. An orderly will be here shortly to bring you to the radiology department. I will check in on you upon your return. And don't worry, we will take good care of you. Now, are you sure you didn't get hurt playing football?"

As I laughed still holding my collarbone in place, I responded, "Let's just say it was football. It will make for a better story."

And then she was gone.

"Thank you for not telling Linda I did this playing whiffle ball."

"Don't worry. I know you too well."

"Mr. Dahlborg, my name is Mike. I'll be wheeling you to x-ray."

"Hi, Mike. Can my wife come too?"

"Absolutely. And no worries. You just relax on this stretcher and I will have you there quick as a whistle."

I thought only my grandfather said, "quick as a whistle." Clearly my mind was trying to focus away from my brokenness as we rolled from the ER to x-ray.

"Here we are," Mike said as he stopped the stretcher against a wall apparently just outside the x-ray waiting area. "The x-ray tech will get you shortly. Then once you are done, they will call me again, and I will come back and get you to bring you back to the ER. Again, no worries."

I must have looked worried.

Mike was very pleasant. He talked just enough. He smiled. He made jokes. He looked me in the eyes. He knew my name. He made sure Doc was with me. He made me feel cared for (just as Linda in the ER had done).

Mike and Linda engaged with me and my bride (my family) the way I hoped I did when I worked in transport years prior and the way I know my bride in her role as a nurse did each day. And together, we engaged with one another. But don't think I wasn't engaged prior to this wonderful connection. I was very much so, as was my wife. We just happened to be blessed to have true caregivers caring for us (and we hadn't even met the doctor yet).

Back in the radiology department, and after a short wait, Barbara, the technologist greeted me and then rolled me into the room for the actual x-ray to take place. Doc was allowed to remain by my side.

"Okay Mr. Dahlberg, to get the picture of your shoulder we will need, I will need for you to hold and then lift a fifteen-pound weight in that left hand. Let me go get the weight. I will be right back."

"Doc, I cannot hold a fifteen-pound weight, never mind lift it. I can't do it," I whispered.

Yes, I have been into fitness all my life. I have played every major sport. I train, workout, and lift weights regularly. But here and now … I am holding my clavicle against my neck and in no way am I going to be able to lift a mere fifteen pounds.

"Don't worry, Tom. Don't worry."

My ability to keep my pain at bay was now waning.

"I cannot do it. I cannot do it. My shoulder won't hold. This is not right. Doc …" I said over and over as Doc looked back at me with those ever-loving eyes.

"Barbara, my husband cannot hold that weight. He is in intense pain. There is no way for him to do what you are asking. Isn't there another way?"

I began to shake as now any control I had had through my mother's magic was lost.

"Please," I was now begging for this healthcare worker to not hurt me. For the system to not harm me. "Please don't ask me to lift that weight."

"This is protocol for this type of injury."

"Ma'am, I know my body. At this time, with this injury, I cannot do it. Please …"

"This is the protocol. I will have to check and get back to you. Excuse me."

With my pain now well over 9 on a scale of 0 to 10 with a ten being the worst, I needed help. I needed someone within the system to care about me.

"Doc …"

And then Linda entered the room.

"Mr. Dahlborg. You will not be lifting any weights today. Don't you worry. We will have pictures of the shoulder taken without any weightlifting. I spoke with the doctor. We are going to take good care of you."

And then leaning close, "Tom, I got you. You are safe."

In my mind I was saying, "Thank you, Linda. You saved me. You understand. You care about me and are caring for me. Thank you. Thank you. Thank you."

But in reality, the tears just built from the intensity of the pain that I was no longer controlling.

Doc however remained in full control.

"Thank you, Linda. Thank you. How will they do the pictures?"

And between the two of them they had it all planned out as to how my shoulder would be x-rayed and where we would go from here.

"Thank you, Doc." I whispered as she held my hand, and I closed my eyes.

The x-rays were completed without any weightlifting. (Please don't tell my buddies at the gym I opted out of moving some weight.)

And then Mike came back to get me and wheel me back to the ER.

"You look none the worse for wear, Tom."

"You have no idea, Mike. Linda and my bride are my heroes."

And with that we arrived back in my bay in the ER.

"Here you go, Tom. You'll be okay. Just listen to Linda and your wife. They will be sure you are taken care of."

"Thank you, Mike."

I wish I had said more. I wish I had said that his words of encouragement meant so much to me even though I was *just* here for a shoulder. I wish I had said that his caring is what healthCARING is all about.

Instead, I simply said, "Thank you, Mike."

Doc and I then waited for another few hours as the results of my films were received by the on-call doctor. But during this time period, Linda stopped by a number of times to thank us for our patience and to let us know we were not forgotten.

Truth be told, I did not feel forgotten with Linda on the case.

"Mr. Dahlborg. I am Dr. Fox. I have reviewed your films. You have a significant separation in that shoulder. We are going to relocate the bone and tape it down. We will then send you home with a recommendation to see your orthopedist. Does that make sense? Are you ready?"

This, I believe, was the first time I completely removed my right hand from my collarbone since the initial injury. And believe it or not, it was hard to do. Not necessarily due to pain or a physical need at this point but rather from the emotional and psychological perspective. "If I let go of this bone it will rip me open," I was thinking. But slowly and carefully, I did let go and surrendered to Dr. Fox and Linda as they set my shoulder and taped me up.

Dr. Fox -- focused and efficient. Linda -- talking to me the whole time. Reassuring me. Both caring about me and yet in different ways.

"You will want to ice this area for 20-30 minutes a few times per day until you see your doctor. I will write you a prescription for the pain, and you will want to take ibuprofen as directed. Do you understand?"

"Yes, doctor. Thanks."

And then, he was gone.

In the meantime, Linda had tracked down a wheelchair.

"Tom, I will help you off of the stretcher and into this chair. First, let me make sure the wheels on each are locked."

Ever vigilante. Ever caring.

"Alright, Darlene, please support Tom near his right shoulder as I support his left arm. Tom, I want you to slowly sit up and begin to turn your body so that your legs are near the edge of the stretcher."

Come on, Mom-magic. I need you again, I remember thinking as I took a deep breath and followed orders.

"That's it. Now use your right hand and support yourself as I guide you to the chair."

Easier said than done for sure.

"That's it. You are there. Now I will place your feet on these two pedals, and we will slowly move toward the door. Darlene, why don't you get your car and drive up to the door to meet us."

"Okay." And then looking me deep in the eyes, "Tom, I'll be right back."

I don't remember getting into the car. And just as with Mike, I don't recall saying thank you or goodbye to Linda. I truly wish I did. (I hope I did.) Linda and my bride truly saved me. Or at least saved me from a great deal of unnecessary pain and harm. The entire healthcare system can learn much by simply watching the Mike's and Linda's do their jobs. And even better, not just watching but rather ensuring we are positioning them, better said, caring about them as they care about their patients.

"Thank you, Linda. Thank you, Mike. Thank you," I whispered to the Universe as Doc drove me home.

"So!"

Uh oh. I am in real trouble, I remember thinking.

"So. You ruined ..."

Yes, I ruined my son's first birthday party, I thought. I am so sorry, *Tommy.*

"... you ruined one of my favorite t-shirts!"

Phew.

"And you ruined the greatest kid's birthday party duck game ever!" Doc continued now laughing that amazing 'brings smiles to ever one's face' laugh.

"I know. I know. I am so sorry."

"You know, and I know that you will never learn. Whether it is pickup basketball, touch football, or whiffle ball at your son's birthday party, you are never going to learn."

And then a deep breath. Probably by both of us.

"I am sorry you are hurt, my love."

"Thank you, Honey. I am sorry I ruined Tommy's party."

By the time we got home, everyone except for my parents (and my children and Angus of course) had gone home.

"Hey, Big T!" I said with as much energy as I could muster. "Hey, Sammy! Did you take care of Tommy while we were away?"

"Daddy, are you okay? I was so scared by the loud siren and seeing you and mommy go away."

"I am so sorry, Sammy. I am fine. Just a little boo boo on my shoulder. Everything is okay now. And me and momma are home."

Nothing like a big hug from a child. Yes, even a hug across a dislocated shoulder. Nothing better.

"Tommy, how'd you make out?"

My mom looked very worried.

"Your magic worked wonders, Mom. I was able to hold the pain off for most of the adventure. The folks at Morton were wonderful, and between them and Doc, I was well taken care of."

"So, what was the diagnosis?"

Dad looked worried too.

"I separated my left shoulder pretty good, Dad. They taped the clavicle down for now and referred me to the orthopedic surgeon."

"Well, you certainly do know how to clear a room."

REFLECTION

In 1992, the American Academy of Pediatrics (AAP) ad-hoc committee on the patient-centered medical home (PCMH) put out a policy statement highlighting, among other key attributes, the importance of compassionate care.

By 2007, a shared group comprised of the AAP, American Academy of Family Physicians, American College of Physicians and American Osteopathic Association developed and shared a statement of joint principles of the medical home, which also noted many of its key attributes.

As I reviewed the evolution of the policy statement and principles I was struck by the fact that by 2007, compassionate care was no longer set as one of the highest priority areas for the PCMH but rather included as a subset under quality and safety.

So why is compassion no longer a key focus of the PCMH?

When I posed this question to an expert in this space, the response and perspective was quite interesting:

> *"Pediatricians have tended to always practice this way, with compassion. As other organizations came to the table and the PCMH concept expanded beyond the pediatric office, more and more weight was placed on the technical aspects of care provision and less and less on compassionate care."*

And when I step back and take a more global view of challenges within the healthcare system, I find the further we move away from a focus on compassion, the further we move away from our ultimate goal and responsibility of ensuring those we are blessed and entrusted to serve are well taken care of and kept safe.

Some examples:

- *We hear more and more about the shortage of primary care physicians and yet we don't create a model of primary care that allows physicians the opportunity to truly connect with their patients, develop relationship and trust, hear whole stories, share empathy, and show compassion, while also having the opportunity to truly connect with their own passion for healing.*

- *We hear more and more about physician burnout and nurses suffering from depression and yet we continue to incentivize with money, continue to focus on productivity, and continue to understaff healthcare organizations (placing our patients and our staff at risk). We continue to move further and further away from our patients and compassionate care provision (while noting "technology will replace human connection") and wonder why we no longer have joy in healing (but rather burnout, depression, and suicide).*
- *We talk more and more about improving health outcomes and doing so efficiently and yet we dismiss the empirical data that supports the view that compassion in healing improves health outcomes.*
- *Physicians pledge to honor the Hippocratic Oath, which includes the statement" ... warmth, sympathy, and understanding may outweigh the surgeon's knife or the chemist's drug." Yet we do not create systems that allow for a focus on warmth and sympathy along with an appropriate balance of surgical, pharmaceutical, technological, and other medical / behavioral interventions.*

The patient-centered medical home and its continued evolution may be a step in the right direction, but we must refocus its principles to ensure compassionate care is elevated in the hierarchy of priorities.

Questions

1. As a healthcare leader, clinician, or staff person, what is your role in engaging patients and families?

    a. How successful are you in this role?

    b. How do you know?

    c. What are keys to your success (best practices)?

2. As a patient or family member, please share a story of a time when you most felt cared for, safe, perhaps even loved within the healthcare system?

    a. Who helped you to feel that way?

    b. What made the difference?

Chapter 22

Shoulder Surgery (1997)

For the next week or so I slept sitting up in a recliner in our living room as we awaited the appointment with the surgeon.

At this time, I was between knee surgeries and in need of a new surgeon. And with Doc having worked at the Harvard Community Health Plan Staff Model health center in Braintree, as well as my primary care physician still being located there, I took their advice and scheduled an appointment with Dr. Athens, an onsite orthopedic surgeon with a good 'cutter' reputation.

On the day of the visit, I was a bit nervous and anxious to move forward with healing as quickly as possible.

"I'm Dr. Athens. You separated your shoulder. Are you a professional athlete?"

I wonder if backyard whiffle ball counts.

"No."

"Then the best course of action is to continue to ice it, take NSAIDs, keep it immobile in the sling for another week, and let me know if it worsens. If it doesn't, we will get you back in to meet with my PA and begin a stretching program. Understood?"

And that was it. In and out in less than seven minutes. Course of action dictated. My job was clear ... follow doctor's orders.

"Doc, Dr. Athens did not recommend surgery."

I was pleased of course that surgery was not necessary at this time, but was also curious as to whether any financial drivers for Dr. Athens had an influence in his decision-making.

"Oh, Tom, if a surgeon is saying 'no surgery,' that is a very good thing."

Over the next few weeks, the pain in my head attributable to my shoulder injury became almost unbearable even as I continued to take my ibuprofen religiously.

And at my next appointment with Dr. Athens, I let him know where things stood.

"Tom. Here is what we can do. We can take a ligament from your left arm and use that to stabilize your shoulder."

"What will that do to my left arm?"

"It will make it less stable."

Didn't sound like a good option to me.

"Or we can do what is known as a clavicle resection where I will cut off the end of the bone to get that now floating bone off of the nerve which, of course, is causing you your headaches."

"Downside?"

"Normal surgical risks. Upside is you should not have the head pain any longer."

"Sounds like we should do it. How soon can we make it happen?"

"You will talk with my scheduler, and she will get you all set. In the meantime, I am writing you a prescription for Naproxen. I want you to take this every day. It will replace the ibuprofen. Got it?"

And a few weeks later I had my clavicle resected, and all went well as far as the surgery itself. I was treated very well at the ambulatory surgical center. The clavicle resection was completed, there was no acquired infection, I was released on the same day and slept in my own recliner (wish I could say bed) that evening.

However, and perhaps most important, the head pain never did decrease, and I continued my daily Naproxen regimen until years later when a new physician prescribed the Vioxx.

REFLECTION

"Honor knows no statute of limitations." - Samuel E. Moffat

I remember not too long ago a discussion with a leader of a prestigious healthcare quality improvement organization:

"Once we have a financial model in place, our ability to improve healthcare provision will be much more attainable."

"It requires a financial model to be in place prior to doing the right thing? We cannot wait. Patients are being wounded. Families are being harmed. Communities are being hurt. Over 50 percent of inpatient adverse events are preventable. The harm rate in healthcare is staggering. Yes, a financial model aligned with our aims is important, but doing the right thing should not be dependent on it. We need to identify those people who truly value patient safety—those people who are not reliant on a new financial incentive to do what is right, those people who truly care—and ensure they are positioned to both lead and serve in an effort to improve the healthcare system. A financial model is important. It is also a technical fix to an adaptive challenge. We cannot wait."

"Tom, I agree. We must do both. I just know that the system will not change until we align the financial drivers."

"And yet the pendulum has swung from fee for service to fee for service with withholds to capitation (primary care cap, specialty cap, contact cap, global cap) to quality-based incentives (now called pay for performance) back to fee for service but now married with P4P models, and so on and so on. And in each instance, maximizing revenues and market share has become a keen focus for many. It has become a game. How about we do what is right first? The opposite has been tried and failed too many times, and too many people have been hurt far too often."

"True. And yet to turn this ship we must get the financing right."

There are a great many people of value, of integrity, and of honor within the healthcare system who strive each and every day to do what is right for patients, families, and communities as well as for doctors, nurses, and staff throughout the system.

These are the people we must engage.

These are the people we must ensure are at the proverbial table, be it the health system board, the leadership teams of the hospitals and medical groups, the local health and/or healthcare non-profits, and so many more.

These are the people who, when the funding model changes, their values do not.

These are the people that when times get tough, they lean in to do what is right rather than bail out and take an easier, more lucrative role.

These are people who are like the many physicians I have been blessed to know who left lucrative practices that "steal their soul" to focus on innovating the healthcare model so that patients and families are truly embraced, whole stories truly heard and honored, and treatment plans co-created and aligned with patient preferences. And have done so even though they are not maximizing their individual revenue.

These are people like the many nurses I have also come to know who don't even take breaks to go to the bathroom as they focus 100% of their daily efforts to care for patients and families, as well as doctors, staff and one another under challenging circumstances at best.

These are people like the physician assistant in Northern Maine who risked her job to find a solution to emergency department overcrowding — which did not include spending limited capital on more bricks and mortar with a goal of financially maximizing ED visits.

Yes, system improvement (i.e., an aligned financial model) is essential to an optimal healthcare model. And yet, at this time, it is not as important as identifying and leveraging those who are both within the system and outside the system who embrace healthCARING values.

We must ensure these individuals are whole and healthy and help position them so that they may lead and serve with great joy using their skills, wisdom, gifts and passions for the betterment of society.

"THE GREATNESS OF A MAN IS NOT IN HOW MUCH WEALTH HE ACQUIRES, BUT IN HIS INTEGRITY AND HIS ABILITY TO AFFECT THOSE AROUND HIM POSITIVELY." - BOB MARLEY

Questions

1. As a patient or family member, how important do you believe are financial drivers to physicians making clinical decisions?

    a. How important should they be?

    b. Do you believe patients and family members should be aware (transparency) of the financial drivers impacting their care decisions? Why or why not?

Chapter 23

Back to the Emergency Room (2001)

After what seemed an eternity in my cell, but now with the love of my life by my side, the nurse rejoined us.

"Mr. Dahlborg, we are having problems finding you a bed on the cardiac floor. If I cannot secure one shortly, we will put you on med/surg. It's not a big deal, but of course we would prefer you on a step down unit. I will be back shortly."

"I am so sorry, dear."

"I should be saying that to you, Doc."

And for the next few hours we remained alone in our cell, together. Our love not spoken with words of the ages (I wish it had been) but rather us both physically, mentally, and emotionally exhausted.

"Doc, the kids are still with Maureen?"

Doc had been on the phone off and on with our new best friend, our realtor Maureen, who was still watching our children as Doc stayed with me.

"Yes, honey. I feel so bad."

Maureen is an older woman who, without warning, had inherited our children for the day.

"Call Maureen back and make plans to get the kids and go home. It makes no sense for you to be spending so much time with me here just waiting."

"I don't want to leave you. What if something happens?" Doc said as a solitary tear rolled down her cheek.

"Just come back and take me home tomorrow."

"Okay, Tom. Okay. It is unfair to Maureen. The kids must be worried. I will get them home."

Asking Doc to leave me and Doc feeling so torn but eventually agreeing to do so for our children (we had no family local and both believed we had already taxed our friends enough) was one of hardest things we each had to do.

"I love you, Tom."

In the movie the Princess Bride, when Wesley and Buttercup finally kiss, it is said of this kiss, "Since the invention of the kiss, there have only been five kisses that were rated the most passionate, the most pure. This one left them all behind."

Our goodbye hug was like that kiss on this day.

"I love you, Doc. I am so sorry."

"Shhhhhh … I will see you tomorrow. No worries. I love you."

As I solitaired for the next few hours in my cell, a feeling of aloneness descended upon me like locusts onto a wheat field. My head, neck, shoulder pain … my chest pain? No … it was this aloneness now that became my tormentor. A crepuscule shroud being manifested now within my chest as the weight of the empty reminded me that not only my better half but my wholeness had left me.

My only refuge was each time I closed my eyes and brought my beautiful children and my loving bride back to me in my dreams.

As the beeps and hums and yells and cries encompassed me, I turned to the faces of the four people I cherished and loved the most to bring the Light of Peace into my soul as the demons of fear and loneliness tried to fight their way into my heart.

"My heart, my chest, I cannot breathe", I yelled, but alas I was dreaming again as the time in my prison cell with its grey flowing walls and intense white lights grew longer.

"Mr. Dahlborg. We have a room for you. We have a room."

> *"Wonderful. We have been waiting here for a long time, and my kids want to get to the pool …"*

"Mr. Dahlborg. Mr. ..."

Slowly I awoke to my nurse sharing the good news.

"You had me nervous, Mr. Dahlborg. You stopped breathing for a moment. I am so glad you are back with us. We have a room for you. You will be on a med/surg floor ... but not to worry, they will keep a close eye and take good care of you."

And then after a brief pause and look around my cell, "Where is Mrs. Dahlborg?"

"My wife went home to be with our children. They were getting nervous."

"Okay. That makes sense." And then putting her hand on my arm for the first time since inserting an IV hours earlier, "They will take great care of you upstairs."

And then as she squeezed my arm, "Transport will be here momentarily. I will also walk up with you to ensure the orders are passed along as the doctor wishes. We will monitor your heart overnight, we will assess your enzymes a couple of more times over the next twelve hours and make sure your heart is stable before sending you home."

Home sounded like heaven.

"Dr. Mewnfrys has also ordered a stress test in the morning so be sure to get some sleep tonight."

A stress test? I was not sure what that was exactly, but did note that the thought of it alone did promote stress.

"Is this Mr. Dahlborg?"

"Yes, Mike. This is Mr. Dahlborg."

Another Mike in transport. *This must be a good sign,* I remember thinking.

"He is going up to the med/surg floor. The cardiac floor is full tonight and short staffed. I will be joining you for the stroll to pass along all the information they will need."

"Sounds great. Tom?"

Tom? Is this the 'Mike' from Morton Hospital all those years ago, and does he remember me?

"I see your name is Tom. Do you mind if I call you that?"

I guess not. But still a good sign.

"That would be great, Mike."

Mike spoke to me the entire way to my floor. I am not sure what he said as I was still floating in and out of the dark, but between him and my nurse there was enough Power of Light for me to hold and embrace.

"Tom, they will take good care of you on this floor." And then he whispered, "By the way, this is my favorite floor. You are in good hands. And if you need anything ask for Linda."

Linda? Another good sign.

"Or if you just want to take a joy ride, you just ask them to page Mike and I will come up and getcha."

Another true healer. And as before, I wished I had told Mike that.

I wish I had said, "Mike, I felt scared and alone. My wife had left to be with our kids. I was afraid I was going to die. I was cold, and this feeling of doom was still creeping in all around me. You have helped me heal. You asking to call me by my first name, you talking with me about the Sea Dogs, about taking a joy ride. You joking with me and not at me. You are a caregiver. I hope you know that. And thinking back to when I was in transport … I hope I was, too. Thank you for caring for me and about me. I feel a little less scared and the darkness of fear was pushed back behind your Light. Thank you."

My nurse spoke with the floor nurses and ensured all my information was transferred accordingly. She then approached me, "Tom," I do like the sound of that. "Linda and the rest of the care team here will take great care of you. Feel better."

And then she was gone.

"Tom, my name is Linda. Mike told me to keep an extra special look out for you."

"He is a good guy."

"Yes, he is."

Now this was a true care team. Linda and Mike truly seemed to care for one another. And now they were each caring for me.

"I will be guiding you into your room in a moment, and then I will help you off of this stretcher and into your bed. Are you going to make it easy for me or will I need to ask for some additional help?" Linda said with a wink.

Smiling and forgetting some more of my fear and loneliness for the moment, I responded, "I think I got this."

When it was time, Linda carefully guided me from the stretcher to the bed while ensuring I did not fall and my IV was not disturbed.

And once in the hospital bed, she reattached the pulse oximeter, the heart monitor feeds, and an automatic blood pressure cuff.

"I am going to have to get a larger cuff for you. Do you lift weights?"

YES! Got to relish the small wins when you can, I figured.

"A little. Back in the day."

I can't believe I just said, 'back in the day'. My parents say back in the day. Was I becoming my dad?

"I can tell. I will get a larger cuff. It will be more comfortable for you, and we will get a more accurate reading."

"Thank you, Linda."

"I will be right back. You relax as best you can. Take natural breaths."

After I watched Linda leave my room, I took a moment to scan my surroundings. The room was bare. There was nothing here except my bed, a small cabinet of some sort next to me, and … whiteness. "Perhaps to combat the darkness," I said to myself.

The room was empty. The room was bright. And the room was cold. Ice cold.

"Tom, how is your head?"

Linda had returned with the larger cuff.

"It is still pounding. I am not sure if it is from the nitro or me missing my Vioxx."

"Why are you on Vioxx? I don't see that in your chart."

"For joint and head pain. I take it daily. Prior to Vioxx I was taking Naproxen."

"Ok. I have the Naproxen listed but not the Vioxx. I will update our chart. In the meantime, I will see what I can do for your head. How is your chest pain?"

"I am okay."

"Listen. Don't try to be a tough guy for me."

If she only knew. If she only knew I just wanted to go home and cry.

"Tom, I need you to be real with me. My job is to take care of you and keep you safe. You need to help me do so. You need to partner with me. Capiche?"

Linda was right. We were supposed to be a team. I have a role. And I must push ego aside and be honest.

"I have never had these types of pains before. So, I am challenged to define a 9 or a 10. I don't know if it can or will get worse."

"You must be an analyst!"

We both chuckled a bit.

"Linda, I have been trying to manage this chest pain and pressure for a couple of weeks. Sometimes it has been so painful that I am not able to stand up. And at other times, it has felt like someone was sitting on my chest … and everything in between. Right now, I am not at the worst. And if that worst is a ten then I would say my pain is currently at a six and the weight on my chest is like an eight."

"Very helpful, Tom. Now tell me about your breathing."

"Since the initial spell, it has been challenging. I feel like my chest can't expand to get a deep breath. I feel like my lungs are only partially filling up. Even just talking with you is challenging."

"And what is this about a broken nose?"

With this, I almost laughed out loud.

"I have no idea. But I do know that the doctor who said that really upset my wife."

"What do you mean?"

"My wife and I were alone in my ER bay when the curtain was pulled back abruptly, and a physician we had never seen before said something like, 'I know why you can't breathe. You have a broken nose.' And then she left as fast as she came. My wife, who is a nurse, was so upset that this person who didn't know us and did not know my story, would barge into our space, not introduce herself, not ask me any questions, not make any effort to connect other than to say 'You broke your nose,' and then just disappear never to be seen by us again."

As Linda nodded, I continued.

"I have been punched in the nose on numerous occasions, been hit in the nose by footballs, basketballs, baseballs, and possibly even a softball, but with all of that I don't ever remember literally breaking my nose. But perhaps I did. I do know I was never seen by a doctor for a broken nose. Is a broken nose now in my medical record?"

Linda shook her head, placed her hand on my hand, and said, "Don't worry about it now. You are in good hands on this floor."

And then …

"I am going to apply some more nitro paste on your chest to help alleviate some of your chest discomfort. This will go right over your coronary arteries to help open them up. Unfortunately, this may exacerbate your headache, but we will manage that."

I replied, "Okay", but I really didn't want this headache to worsen.

With great care, Linda loaded the paste onto what looked like parchment paper and then placed it on my chest over my heart.

"Your chest will feel better shortly. I am also going to give you oxygen to take some stress off of your lungs."

And with that she placed a clear hose around my head and inserted two mini tubes from the hose into my nostrils.

"Just breathe normal. This will help."

It was now looking like I am really sick for sure.

"I will get you some ice water. This container here is for you to urinate in. If you need to have a bowel movement, just press this black button. If you need anything, just press that button."

I must have looked stressed again.

"Tom, I got you. I am here."

REFLECTION

Years later, I would be meeting with senior leaders from one of the most prestigious medical systems in the country, renowned for its focus on patient experience and empathy, and they would ask me about patient experience in an inpatient setting.

I, of course, reflected back to the Mike's in transport at both Morton and Mercy Hospital, and of Linda in the Emergency Room at Morton and on the med/surg floor at Mercy, and I would share the impact each of these people had on my experience as a patient and the feeling I had that I was truly care about.

I would continue by sharing my own experience working in transport at Brockton Hospital where I had the opportunity to talk with many patients and their families as we walked together to radiation oncology, physical therapy, x-ray, and many other departments. And how I hoped that our discussions impacted these people as much as Mike and Linda impacted me.

And lastly, I talked about a good friend who was in the hospital over an Easter weekend and how she shared a story with me about how alone she felt on that Sunday morning when a custodian came in, smiled, and handed her a stuffed bunny. And to this day, that is her positive patient experience memory from her hospital stay.

And the response from these senior leaders?

> *"But what about HCAHPS?"*

When people talk about patient engagement, patient activation, and patient experience, many times the focus is on numbers and the specific impact of doctors and nurses. And clearly this is very important (especially the clinician impact). And yet, all of us working in healthcare have the opportunity to engage, to connect, to care, and to love those we work with and those patients and families we serve. We must expand our minds to truly serve and impact.

Questions

1. As a healthcare leader or nurse, what is the optimal nurse-to-patient ratio in the emergency room? On a med/surg floor in a hospital?

    a. How do you know?

2. As a healthcare leader, how do you ensure nurses are best positioned to provide person- centered care?

3. As an emergency room nurse, please describe a typical day, your focus, your challenges, your goals, and barriers to achieve your goals?

4. As an emergency room physician, please describe a typical day, your focus, your challenges, your goals, and barriers to achieve your goals?

5. As a patient or family member, please share your story of a recent visit to the emergency room. The positive encounters and impacts as well as the challenges you faced.

    a. Did you feel listened to?

    b. Did you feel cared for?

    c. Did you feel safe?

    d. Did you feel loved?

Chapter 24

Mercy Hospital

"Tom. Tom. I need you to wake up. We need to draw more blood to measure your cardiac enzymes again. This is Maria. She will be drawing your blood."

"What time is it?"

"It's about 1:00am. How is your head?"

"How did you know? It's still pounding."

"I'll get you something for that."

"You were thrashing about. Were you having a nightmare?"

I believe Linda was trying to take my mind off of the phlebotomist inserting what appeared to be the longest needle ever into my right arm.

"Actually I was. I was dreaming about my internship at a world renowned hospital in Massachusetts. The people there were very nice and all, but the department was completely dysfunctional. I was dreaming about the waste and harm."

"That sounds intense."

"It was really challenging being there. I felt like I had no power or control. I felt like I didn't contribute as much as I could have. And I felt like I wasn't learning much. Basically, wasting my time and my education."

"All set, Mr. Dahlstrom."

"Thank you," I said to the phlebotomist as she finished up and carried my blood away.

"What did you do?" Linda asked. I believe she was truly interested.

"I thought long and hard about my experience and what I was not getting from it. And then I realized, actually I was learning a great deal. I was learning the "how nots." How not to run a department. How not to engage. How not to be efficient and effective. How not to honor a mission. And that is what I wrote my paper about, and that is what I shared in class."

"It actually sounds like an amazing experience when you put it that way."

"It really was. I learned so much that I have carried with me to this day. The "how nots." Maybe I'll write a book about it one day?" I joked.

"That would be a great book."

Linda really seemed to care about me as a patient. And as a person. Even at 1:00am.

"How is your chest pain on a scale of 1 to 10 with ten being the worst?"

"It is at a seven as far as the pressure on my chest. And a six as far as actual pain."

"Okay. I am going to give you another nitroglycerin tablet and will check the paste. Don't worry we will get you comfortable."

Linda looked at the paste and then took my blood pressure. She checked all of my tubing and then laid her hand on my head and looked me in the eyes as she said, "Try to sleep now. I am here if you need me."

Doc and I have these feelings that we call "warm fuzzies." She will say, "Honey, I just got this warm fuzzy feeling about you." And then a hug. Or I will call her from the car and say, "Doc, I just got that warm fuzzy again. I love you. Can't wait to see you and hold you tonight."

We have discussed these warm fuzzies a great deal and have arrived at the belief that this is when God reaches in to send us a reminder of our love for one another. The feeling we each have (usually at differing times) is of an overwhelming presence of love sweeping through each cell of our body and touching both our heart and our soul. Many times, I know the feeling will prompt a tear or two as this Love takes hold and the world takes a step back.

And even with Linda by my side, this night I needed that warm fuzzy.

By 3:00am the pain in my head swelled to well beyond a ten (if that is even possible), as did the pain and Giles Corey pressure on my chest, and my body began to tremble.

"Please God get me through this night. I promise I will do anything you ask," I remember pleading. "Please let me hold my bride and my children once again. Even just once more."

I have read there are no atheists in foxholes. I wonder how many people beg, plead, and negotiate with the Universe on nights such as this.

Why is it so dark here? I thought. *And who is that. I cannot see. Are those footsteps?*

I listened more intently.

Yes, they were. Getting closer and closer. Louder. Louder. Again, I called out, *Who is that?*

"Mr. Dahlberg. You are dreaming, Mr. Dahlberg. I need you to relax. Your heart rate is through the roof."

As I slowly began to exit my dream, I saw a new nurse looking down upon me.

"Breathe, Mr. Dahlberg. Breathe."

I can't breathe. My chest feels like it has an elephant standing on it.

"Take a slow deep breath, Mr. Dahlberg. I need you to relax. You can do it." And as she held my right hand, "I am right here with you. My name is Nancy. I'll be taking care of you this morning. Now give me a deep breath."

"I can't Nancy. My diaphragm feels like it is stuck in cement. And I can't breathe out of my nose."

"What is your pain level from 1 to 10 with ten being the worst?"

"The pressure on my chest is a ten. My head pain is an eight. My chest pain is as well."

"Let's see what we can do to help you get comfortable."

And then, a calming smile.

Thank you. Thank you for looking me in the eyes. Thank you for seeing me, I responded but only in my head.

A few hours later after some tweaking of positions, more nitro pills, and something for my head I was feeling a bit better and ready to call Doc. I wanted her with me so very badly and yet part of me was pushing for her to stay home. Being seen so broken and ready to break down at any moment was not how I really wanted to present myself.

"Doc, it's Tom."

"I know who it is. I'll be there within the hour. How are you?"

"I am scared, baby."

"I know. Me, too. I will be there shortly. I love you."

I then looked upward and began to pray again …

"There is no way this is a heart attack. There is no way I am not going home today. God, we talked it over last night. I'll be honest. I don't remember where we left off. But this I know … we got this. You and me. Option 1, I've got the flu. Option 2, I got something going on with my heart. But we got this. My wife is a nurse, I've been working in healthcare in one way or another since 1984, so that is seventeen years. I've been working in Maine for 1.5 years, but in that time I have developed relationships and now have contacts with many prominent healthcare leaders … if I need a cardiologist I know the head of Vascular Associates, if I need to be hospitalized again I know many leaders within both Maine Med and Mercy. I've got this. We've got this. You in, God? I am not dying today."

If only this was just another football game.

I was getting all worked up, and my monitor was going kind of crazy again.

Nancy is not going to like this.

In my mind I began to make a list. "Cardiology. Ok. I know Jerry Schmidt. He is the lead guy. Check."

I continued through primary care, other specialists, and hospital contacts until my head pounded even worse. And then finally, "Saul. My boss Saul knows everybody. If I need anyone else, he should be able to direct me. Check."

"Okay. I got this. Bring it on!"

The false or at least denial-based bravado was working in full force.

"Mr. Dahlborg. Dr. Mewnfrys will be up shortly. He has scheduled you for a stress test this morning. He also wants to check in on your breathing. Your ER notes mention a broken nose and much difficulty breathing."

"I didn't break my nose. At least not recently and never diagnosed."

"Okay. The doctor will be up within the hour and you can work that all out. Can I get you anything?"

"An eraser to erase the note about my broken nose?"

Nancy laughed. But I wasn't kidding. How did a "broken nose" get added to my chart with no examination of it other than one physician in the ER who did not know me, did not talk with me, and did not examine me other than from across my cell? And what is the process to clean my record? I wondered how often this happens. In this case. it is more of a pain in the butt. But what about real mix ups?

"Seriously, is there a way to fix my medical record? I do not have a broken nose. And I was not admitted to the ER or overnight to the med/surg floor for a broken nose."

"You will need to discuss that with Dr. Mewnfrys. But for now, don't worry about it. It's not a big deal."

Maybe not a big deal in my case. But what about other situations? Inaccurate medical information input into someone's medical record could be very dangerous and a very big deal.

"Mr. Dahlborg, nice to see you again. I am Dr. Mewnfrys. How are you feeling this morning?"

"I am still feeling the chest pain and pressure. And now I have a pounding headache either from the Nitro or because I still haven't had my Vioxx."

"Nurse, please get me Mr. Dahlborg's chart."

"Right away, Doctor."

"I have you booked for a stress test this morning."

"Here is his chart."

And then, after what appeared to be an hour, "Good news Mr. Dahlborg. Your cardiac enzymes have not elevated over the past twelve hours."

"Tell me about your breathing."

"It has been a bit of a struggle over the last couple of weeks. Tough to get a deep breath. Sometimes it feels like I cannot expand my ribcage."

"I noticed in the ER some wheezing. How long has this been going on?"

"Well, the difficulty breathing has been about two weeks."

"Okay. I am going to write you a couple of prescriptions for your breathing to help open you up. One is a quick acting inhaled steroid bronchial dilator to address any urgent need and the other is a maintenance dilator I will want you to take daily."

Two things came to mind immediately. *I wish Doc was here to explain these things to me. I don't like taking anything and have never needed an inhaler before.* And the other was, *A steroid? Some of my boys in Brockton would be drooling at the thought.*

"Your CT for a possible PE came back negative."

My what for a what is what? was all I could think.

"I don't know what that means."

"Your CAT scan last evening for a possible pulmonary embolism came back negative."

I still had no idea what he is talking about and didn't recall having a CT scan last evening.

"Good morning, Honey."

Thank God. Doc is here.

"Hi Honey. This is Dr. Mewnfrys."

"Hi Doctor. I am Tom's wife, Darlene. I remember you from yesterday."

"Good morning. I was just sharing with him that his enzymes have leveled off, his CT scan for a PE is negative, and for his breathing I am prescribing a couple of bronchial dilators."

"He was diagnosed with sports-induced asthma years ago," [I was?], "but was not prescribed an inhaler at that time."

"He will have a stress test this morning and, depending on the outcome, I will determine next steps. Okay?"

I assumed Dr. Mewnfrys did not hear Doc's comment about the sports-induced asthma.

"Yes, doctor."

"Question, why do you think his cardiac enzymes were elevated?"

Leave it to Doc to go right at it.

"He has had damage to his heart. Possibly a heart attack."

"A heart attack. Okay. Next steps?"

"Stress test this morning. If negative, we send him home and he follows up with his primary care physician and a cardiologist."

"Okay, doctor."

"Doctor, will this be a nuclear stress test?"

"No. Not necessary at this stage of the game." And then turning to me, "Transport will be up shortly to bring you down for the test."

And a few hours later I was transported for my non-nuclear stress test, the test goes off without a hitch, and my results were negative.

(By the way, and I know there are many jokes on TV about this, still when I hear that medical results are negative, I have to think twice to ensure that I am grasping that negative is a good thing. Perhaps we can change the word? Words are quite powerful.)

"Tom, your enzymes are holding steady, your stress test was negative, and you have your two prescriptions for the bronchial dilators. I am going to discharge you, and you will want to follow up with your primary care physician and cardiologist as soon as possible. And, of course, if your chest discomfort worsens you should go to the emergency room immediately."

"Did I have a heart attack?"

"Test results show damage to your heart muscle."

"But did I have a heart attack?"

"You will want to follow up with your primary care physician. But call us if things worsen."

REFLECTION

Even though the stress test has a low sensitivity and specificity, it is noninvasive and inexpensive and is the most common noninvasive test to determine a prognosis in patients with suspected coronary disease.

Interestingly when Dr. Mewnfrys and Doc were discussing my test, my mind at that time did not go to "what if my damaged heart leads to something tragic on the treadmill?" Rather it went back to the year prior to this episode when I was analyzing utilization data for our military healthcare program.

Medical costs in the Bangor market on a per member per month basis were much higher than any other geographic region in the state of Maine for our program. And as my team and I assessed these data and did a root cause analysis (RCA), we discovered a number of interesting things.

First, the gap between medical expense in the different markets was primarily on the outpatient side. This was interesting for a number of reasons including the fact that one of our oldest and more established relationships in the market was with a large primary care group practice, that based on Saul's perspective provided high quality appropriate care. Or as Saul would say, "they know better."

Second, as we continued to drill down using the RCA process, the fishbone diagram and the "five whys," we identified a major driver of the costs in this market was in cardiac testing.

Third, we identified that the number of patients in the Bangor market diagnosed with cardiac disease was comparable to other markets.

Fourth, we also noted that the number of cardiac tests performed in this market were comparable to other markets.

But the two kickers we realized were: 1.) the utilization rate of a nuclear stress test for cardiac testing in the market was substantially higher than all other markets, and 2.) our medical team and quality department noted that the quality of care in the Bangor market was not improved due to the use of the nuclear stress test.

And finally, we determined that the major driver for the use of the nuclear stress test was the fact that a local Bangor practice had invested a large sum of money in this technology.

Again, our quality department determined that the care was not better and, in fact, that our patients (our military members) were being put in harm's way due to exposure to unnecessary radiation that goes along with using the nuclear stress test all because a practice invested in this technology rather than the test was the appropriate healthcare service at the appropriate time for the appropriate person.

Shocking? Unfortunately, no. And, in fact, reminded me of a quote I heard while at Harvard Community Health Plan years prior, "Medical practices will modify how they practice based on compensation models. If we pay according to a fee for service methodology, the number of visits per patient will increase. If we pay according to a primary care capitation methodology, the number of visits per patient will decrease." And in this case, "If a site invests in an ancillary service and we pay according to a fee for service methodology, the utilization of those ancillary services will increase."

Yes, that is where my mind went when talk of my own stress test heated up. Not necessarily a bad thing because at least for a few moments I was not stressing about my potentially literally broken heart.

Plus ... this would further my thinking relative to overtreatment, unnecessary care, financial drivers to care provision, and so much more for years to come.

Questions

1. As a healthcare leader, clinician, staff person, patient, or family member, do you believe money drives medical decisions?

    a. Have you seen instances where money and different payment models have driven a medical decision? Was there a positive or negative impact to the patient?

    b. What would you recommend to improve the system and eliminate or at least limit the financial side of healthcare dictating how care is provided?

Chapter 25

For Everything

"Let me help you into the van."

"Honey, I am okay. They are wrong. I just have the flu."

"Tom ... "

And then silence.

"I am going to get you home and settled. And then I am going to get your prescriptions. They will help you breathe. Then you will feel better."

"What are we doing about my broken nose?"

Darn it. Shouldn't have said that, I scolded myself.

"I am kidding, my love," I said as a new wave of pressure on my chest hit, and I doubled over almost passing out.

"Oh Tom. Look at you. Should we go back to the ER?"

"No. Please just take me home. I just want to get home."

I had forgotten how beautiful the Scarborough marshes are just off of Route One.

The marsh was extra beautiful this day. The herbaceous plant life was almost pink to me. The waterway a deep blue. A number of birds including what looked like double-crested cormorants were standing at attention with their wings spread waving us home. So beautiful. So inviting.

"Almost there."

"Okay dear," I tried to say but couldn't fill my lungs with enough air to do so.

Doc was silent now as we turned left onto Old Blue Point Road.

I wondered what she was thinking as I looked over at the love of my life biting the inside of her cheek. (It is never a good sign when Doc bites the inside of her cheek. This is definitely her 'tell' (as they would say in the movie "Rounders."))

We then turn left on Ryefield Drive. Our street. The street where our home is. Where my children are. Where my puppy is.

A few moments later, Hope has heard us and was opening the door.

"Darlene, you are home. You and Tom are home. Come on in. Come on in. The kids have been wonderful. I am so glad you are home, Tom."

Hope was so kind. And had such an incredible smile. Truly a blessing to us.

"Thank you, Hope."

"The kids have had lunch. Haylee is napping. Tommy is playing upstairs in his room. I hope it is okay. He wanted to stay in his Superman pajamas. He clearly loves running around the house with his cape flying behind him. And Sammy has been such a big helper. She helped pick up after lunch and is now brushing her dolly's hair."

"You are so good, Hope. Thank you so very much."

"Oh, you are welcome, Darlene. But let me get out of the way so you can get Tom settled. Call me if you need anything."

And then shortly after getting settled on the couch …

"Daddy!!!!!"

"Tommy!"

And then with a Superman sonic boom and crash "I love you, Daddy!" Tommy yells as he nearly knocks me over.

"I love you too, Superman."

"Look at my Spiderman motorcycle!"

"Daddy!" I love how Sammy says that. Especially today. "I've missed you. Are you okay?"

"My Sammy. I am fine now that I am home with you."

"Oh shoot. I should have asked Hope to stay longer so that I could get your prescriptions."

"That's okay. I don't need them."

"Listen. Stop. You do need them. I will get them. Not another word."

"Okay. Okay. How about we wait until tomorrow? For now, please just sit with me. That is all I need right now."

"Daddy!!"

"Big T! Come and sit with me."

"I have missed you, dad."

"I've missed you, too. So much."

"Did you really break your heart?"

Out of the mouths of babes.

"Just a little boo boo, T. But now that I am home with you, I am much better."

"I love you, Daddy."

"Can I have a hug?"

"Yes, Daddy!"

"Hey! Sammy and I want in too."

"Thank you, baby."

"For what?"

"For everything."

REFLECTION

I have learned over the years that "bumper sticker" sayings may catch attention and yet without a solid foundation and understanding actually have little impact.

For example: Many of us in healthcare tout the importance of patient and family activation and engagement and yet ...

Each of our patients (each of us) are complex adaptive systems as is each of our family units.

And:

1. *A patient's activation and engagement will vary over time (and perhaps from visit to visit) based on many factors. One example is a patient who may be 100 percent activated and engaged in their own care at their most recent appointment who has learned just after this visit that their parent is now seriously ill and requiring significant support. The next time this patient is seen, the level of activation and engagement may significantly decrease due to such factors as stress, worry, exhaustion, etc. Continuing to assume that the patient is activated at the previous level (based on the most recent visit and data points) will be detrimental to the patient's health and healthcare outcomes.*

2. *To truly provide person-centered care, providers must understand the patient's whole (and ever-evolving) story. What was true last week may have changed significantly and thus no longer holds true, as well as the patient's level of activation and engagement.*

3. *Person centered care includes determining what a specific patient needs at that specific time and not assuming, not strictly relying on tools and not focusing exclusively on data points previously inserted into an electronic health record. Person centered care requires truly and authentically connecting with the patient at each and every healthcare encounter as things change.*

4. *Person centered care recognizes that each patient is different and so is each patient's optimal level of activation and engagement. What is true for "most" patients or even an "average" patient may not be true for the patient sitting in front of you, and it is our responsibility to determine their truth (and also recognizing their truth will change).*

5. *Person centered care recognizes that each patient's family is also different and ever evolving. One person's family may be healthy and whole and a wonderful support, while another's just the opposite. And this will change over time.*

As healthcare leaders, our responsibility is to develop care models that allow for true person-centered care.

We then must create models which position us to modify care and engagement approaches informed by these data.

Questions

1. As a healthcare leader, clinician, or staff person, how reliant are you on patient activation data? How static are these data? How do you know if reliance on these data is truly helpful?

2. As a patient or family member, please describe how engaged and activated you are in your own care? In the care of a loved one? And also, please share what types of scenarios impact your ability to be activated and engaged?

3. What would you recommend to improve or replace measures such as patient activation and patient engagement metrics?

Chapter 26

The Couch

Later that evening with the children fast asleep, Doc and I were alone on the couch together.

"We are going to get you better. I have called Dr. Iuvenis's office, and you have an appointment with him in two days."

Dr. Iuvenis was my current primary care physician. A very nice new doctor. New to my organization and new to practice. He was my second or third primary care physician since I arrived in Maine eighteen months prior. Many physicians had left practice for a variety of reasons. One of those reasons was the productivity requirement placed on them by most practices in order to generate maximum revenue for the practice or hospital system. These caring physicians were burning out and worse.

"We will also get you to the best cardiologist to see what is going on with that big beautiful heart of yours."

"Listen, I just have the flu."

"No, you listen!"

With the sound of Frank Sinatra playing in the background, the love of my life and I fell asleep on the couch and in each other's arms … with are hearts beating as one and our worries at bay for at least a little while.

I love you, my angel, I recall thinking as my bride's inner and outer warmth held me close. *I am so sorry I am putting you through this. I have always wanted to protect you. From any harm I have wanted to protect you, and here I am scaring you. This is not how our adventure to Maine was supposed to play out.*

And then feeling Doc's warmth, my mind became soft again as my bride's breath warmed my cheek.

I do so love holding you. More than anything, I love holding you. You in my arms right now brings me hope and courage. And as we hold one another, I promise ... I will keep you safe ... and I will do whatever it takes to heal. I promise.

REFLECTION

Productivity for physicians is measured in RVUs. An RVU is a relative value unit. Relative value units are one of the key components of the RBRVS system of payment used by Medicare at this time. RBRVS stands for the Resource Based Relative Value System. Other key components of this payment system include the physician's work (the time and skill required for a given procedure), practice expenses (the staff time and costs of maintaining an office), and malpractice expenses. There is also a Geographic Adjustment Factor (GAF), Conversion Factor, "facility" and "non-facility" aspects and other machinations all used to determine how much to reimburse a physician for a service provided to a patient.

That all said, to put it in laymen's terms ... one RVU (again Relative Value Unit) equates to let's call it an "average" office visit between a patient and a physician. And to determine how much that office visit is worth all the components mentioned above are factored in and voila a dollar figure (fee) is determined.

Of note, typically the more invasive a procedure a physician performs the greater the fee. The less invasive the lesser the fee. So, there is a financial incentive to perform not only more procedures but more invasive procedures than other options that may be more appropriate for a specific patient. Now does this mean a physician or administrator may choose to perform an invasive procedure over a non-invasive procedure due to the financial incentive? Actually ... yes. That is the case.

Be it conscious or not that is the case. Clearly not all the time, as I have seen with my many knee injuries where I have been blessed to have found wonderful and caring surgeons who did not always opt for the knife. But that said, I have also found others that have. So this is an area where a patient and family must do their own homework which may mean getting a second and third opinion, and a patient advocate or patient and family advisor who also can be very helpful in ensuring that the patient has all the information they need to make an informed decision.

That all said, many primary care physicians at this time by contract with the practice group or hospital that employs them are obligated to generate a minimum number of RVUs per day. So as an example, if that number is 30 RVUs, that would mean that in a seven-

hour work day, for a primary care physician to achieve this minimum productivity goal, if they were to only schedule "average" office visits, they would need to schedule more than four of these visits per hour. (And that is if they are truly scheduling back to back to back to back visits without the time to review the patient chart, talk with the nurse, and optimally prepare). And based on my experiences and the stories many physicians have shared with me, many are tripled booked every fifteen minutes to ensure revenue is optimized.

So, it is no surprise that many primary care physicians (and nurses) have left their practice and/or left medicine in general. And quite frankly many are not becoming primary care physicians in the first place for this and many other reasons.

These productively requirements move them away from their true calling of caring for their patients. And again, as many have shared, they now must focus on how quickly they determine diagnosis and turf the patient (for example: refer to specialist or prescribe medication) rather than providing the best care possible.

And we wonder why there is a shortage of primary care physicians in America?

Questions

1. As a healthcare leader, clinician, staff person, patient or family member, please share ideas to address the shortage of primary care physicians in America?

2. As a clinician, please share the impact of the current productivity requirements on patient care, safety, engagement as well as on your own well-being.

3. As a patient or family member, how do you believe the current productivity requirements of your clinicians have impacted your care, safety, engagement and well-being?

4. What other healthcare financial models would you recommend to improve the system and why?

Chapter 27

Out of the Mouth of Babes

"Tom, we are going to see Dr. Iuvenis tomorrow morning. He can see you at 10:15am."

Momma Bear was definitely in charge.

Getting an appointment with my doctor was not easy. Open access schedules were still in their infancy and, even though I had had a cardiac event, we could not get in immediately.

"Daddy, I will hold your hand when the doctor talks to you. Mommy always holds me so I am not scared, so I will hold you too."

My heart broke every time I thought of my children seeing their father weak and scared (no matter how I tried to hide it).

"God, this is not supposed to be. I want to be strong. I want my children to see their daddy as invincible. I can't be sick!" I would scream to the All Mighty as my vulnerability exploded into full view for all to see.

"Sammy, you are my angel. Daddy will be fine."

Then after thinking very carefully, or as carefully as I could under the circumstances, "And I would love you to hold my hand with the doctor. How about we hold each other?"

"That sounds perfect, daddy."

"I want to hold you too, daddy!"

"You got it, Big T. We will all hold each other. I am sure Dr. Iuvenis will be fine with that. Cool?"

"Yeah, Dad!" Tommy responded as he ran out of the room to find another adventure for Spiderman and his yellow dinosaurs.

"Dad, I think Tommy just wanted to get in on my action."

Again, out of the mouths of babes.

"Get in on your action, Sam? Where did you learn that?"

"From watching Star Trek with you. You said your favorite episode was 'A Piece of the Action.' Well I think Tommy just wanted in on MY action. I want to hold you. I want to!"

"I am the luckiest man in the world," I thought as I pictured Lou Gehrig at Yankee Stadium all those years ago.

Sammy, you are amazing. You make my heart smile. You have no idea how happy you make me.

"Daddy?"

"Yes, Sam."

"Want to play 'Pretty Pretty Princess' with me?"

"Yes, Sam. Yes. More than anything I want to play 'Pretty Pretty Princess' with you."

Later that evening when I was all alone, I began to pray again.

"God, I would be on my knees if I thought I could get back up on the couch by myself. I am sorry about that. I am scared, God. I am really scared. My breathing is still hard. My chest still hurts. I am exhausted and cannot even get up the stairs to join my wife in bed. My kids are now taking care of me …" I continued as I laid alone on the couch in the dark holding back tears as my worst fears flowed. "This is not right, God. This is not right. I know. I know. The real question is not 'why me?' but rather 'why not me? I know it logically. But … "

"Tom. You were breathing really heavy. Are you okay?"

"Yes. I am okay now. I was just having a dream."

"Well, it is 8:00am. You need to begin to get ready to go to the doctor."

"Sammy and Tommy want to come with me. They want to hold me like you hold them during their doctor appointments."

"They will be in school," and then, seeing the disappointment in my eyes, Doc added, "but Haylee will be with us. She will hold you."

"That will be nice, but I will need to talk to Sam. I totally wasn't thinking. I hope she will understand."

"Sammy. Please come sit next to daddy on the couch," I called out.

"Okay, Daddy."

Sammy looked so beautiful with a sparkle in her blue eyes and her big 'room-brightening' smile.

"Daddy, do you like my hair? I brushed it 100 times this morning. Isn't it pretty?"

"Beautiful, Sammy. Absolutely beautiful," I responded as I also begin a dry coughing fit.

"Daddy, are you okay?"

"Yes. Sammy. When you are next to me, I am always okay."

"You don't sound okay."

Ugh.

"Sammy, I need to see the doctor this morning."

"But I will be in school. How am I going to hold you?"

"That is what I wanted to talk to you about. I need a favor, and I hope you will be okay with it."

"What is it?"

"You know how we pray to Jesus at church and before eating dinner as a family?"

"We don't always pray before dinner."

Once again, out of the mouths of babes.

"I know. We should, but you are right. We don't always. I promise to do better."

"Okay."

Brockton-tough just like her mother, I thought.

"Anyway. Because this time when I see the doctor you and Tommy will be in school, I was hoping that if you remembered, while at school, and only as long as you don't get in trouble, you would find a moment and quietly pray for me. That way even though you won't be holding my hand physically, I will still feel your love around me. Would that be okay?"

"Oh Dad! That is easy. And even if I get in trouble, I will do it."

Uh oh … perhaps a sign of things to come.

"Thank you, Sammy. So, you will be okay not being with me?"

"I want to be with you, but I get it."

"I love you my Sam Bam."

"I love you. Did you tell Tommy yet?"

"He is next."

"I bet he doesn't even remember. Ya know, he was pretty focused on his dinosaurs."

"We shall see. Now go get your breakfast."

"Big T, come here, bud."

Watching Superboy 'fly' across the room with his blond locks, red cape flowing behind him and his big smile is a joy I never want to forget. Actually, more a young Thor than Superboy but then again, he is more DC than Marvel.

"DADDY!!!!!!"

Well, joyful until his head and shoulder crash into my chest ala Tedy Bruschi of the Patriots.

Ugh! Cough Cough Cough

"Big T. I need to go to the doctors this morning while you are in school."

"Okay, Daddy. I'm gonna miss ya."

"I'm gonna miss ya, too. But I am going to think of you the entire time I am there."

"I know, Daddy. And I am going to think of holding your hand while I am in school."

He remembered. He really remembered.

And as tears well up in my eyes, "Thank you, Tommy. You just made my day."

Cough Cough Cough

"Now go get your breakfast. I love you."

"Love you, Dad."

"God, he hits hard, Doc. I think Tommy is going to be a linebacker for the Patriots."

"You just save your breath. This is your first venture out of the house in a long time. You need to save your lungs."

REFLECTION

There is great emotion in healthcare. This is life and death. Life-changing. Yes, emotions are involved. No way around it.

And we should not want there to be a "way around it".

We need to listen to all voices:

- *The voice of the physician who was abused in medical school and has considered taking his or her own life.*
- *The voice of the nurse who is overworked, understaffed and burnt out.*
- *And yes, the voice of the patient who feels scared, alone, frustrated, lost, hopeless.*

And in each case emotions may be involved. In fact, will be involved.

We cannot shy away from it.

We must lean in. We must be vulnerable. And we must be brave. For one another.

Questions

1. As a clinician, patient or family member, is understanding the emotional aspects of illness and the healing process important to you? Why or why not?

    a. If important, how do you address the emotional aspect of illness and the healing process?

    b. What tools do you recommend to ensure the emotional aspects within the healthcare system are honored and addressed?

Chapter 28

The Birds

"Are you ready for this?"

"It is nice to get out of the house," I began. And then add, "And it will be great to hear that this flu is getting better."

Cough Cough Cough

"You know you drive me crazy, don't you?"

"Would you have it any other way, my love?"

I am not sure why I said what I did. Was it just fear of what this might be? Or just downright denial? Or some ego-related thing? All I knew at that point was that I was both very scared and at the same time not willing to believe I was really sick. Both. And.

The ride to see Dr. Iuvenis was fairly quiet. The radio was off, which was unlike us.

The traffic on Route One was flowing well as we headed north past Dunkin Donuts, Len Libby's, and Angus' vet. By the way, Len Libby's has the best chocolate in Maine … and a wicked big chocolate Moose.

As we began to bear off of Route One toward Interstate 295, I noticed a large crow and two smaller birds flying nearby. Apparently racing us.

"Daddy, look at the black birds," Haylee said from the safety of her car seat. "Why is one chasing the other?"

Actually, Haylee was right. They were not racing us. Rather, the two smaller birds were chasing the black crow and periodically attacking.

"Daddy, why is that little bird biting the bigger bird?"

"I am guessing the little birds are mad at the bigger bird for some reason. Maybe he ate their food," I replied to Haylee as I turned to see her all dressed up wearing her favorite pale yellow and light blue 'Holly Hobby' hat. (At least that is what it reminded me of, the Holly Hobby of days gone by that my sister Beanie used to play with.)

"I don't like them fighting."

"I don't either, Haylee. But sometimes even if you're smaller and weaker, you have to stand up for yourself."

"Well, I still don't like them fighting."

I continued to watch the epic battle rage on as we merged onto 295 North toward Exit 9 and Dr. Iuvenis's office.

"Daddy, I think the little birds are very afraid of the bigger bird. But I don't think he did anything wrong. I think they are just scared."

Brockton-tough and wicked smart. Yup, that is my girl, I said to myself. And then to Haylee, "I think you are right, Haylee. Sometimes when we get scared, we act differently than when we feel brave. Sometimes we yell or cry or try to hurt someone else."

"That is not very nice, Daddy."

"I know, Baby. I know. How do you think we could help those little birds to not be scared anymore?"

"I wonder if they are afraid because they are a mommy and daddy, and they are scared that their babies might get hurt by the big bird."

"I bet you are right, Honey. What would you do to help them?"

"If they would listen to me, I would tell them that the big bird looks scary but is really nice. And I would have them play together. First, just the parents. But when they were all friends, I would have the baby birds meet the big bird too."

God, she is smart, I thought.

"I think being scared is okay, Daddy. But I also think that we need to be nice even when we are scared. If the birds would be nice then the scary goes away. Right?"

Cough Cough Cough

"I think you are right, Haylee. Even when we are scared, we should try to focus on being nice. We should try to focus on love. I think if the birds did that then they could stop being afraid. And I think they could even help each other."

"Yeah, Daddy. Yeah …" and then she was quiet for a few moments before finishing, "I love you, Daddy. And I don't want you to be scared."

REFLECTION

Over the years I have found storytelling and poetry to be a pathway for me toward mindfulness and meditation.

Haylee finding meaning in the interaction of the three birds at such a young age continues to inspire me in this space and to this day.

In this realm, I was blessed to have my poem "Birthing Healthcaring" (shared below) featured at a recent Texas gerontology society meeting:

Heart in bay eight?
Knee in room five?
Don't you know who I am?
Don't you know I'm alive?

Look at me I pray
Gaze up from your PC's
Afraid and scared I be today
My heart breaking, down on my knees

I see you are pressed
Rushed and chagrined
Please help me, so stressed
Stop the whirlwind

Lost your soul for healing
Broken system impacts all
I understand your feeling
Passing patients around like a ball

Patient harm as you juggle
A third will be hurt
We ache as you struggle
Our eyes can't avert

Together we must fix
Fanning the flames of care
No more mortar no bricks
Our hearts loaded to bear

Shining light in the darkness
Collaborate and adapt
Serve together and harness
With our love we will craft

Our community we honor
Arising in glory giving
Each patient voice donor
All in service forgiving

We will improve care
Boldly not fearing
A HEARTchange we will dare
Together birthing healthCARING

Questions

1. As a clinician, what does selfcare look like for you? What are your stress relievers?

    a. How has it changed over time?

    b. Do you feel supported in your focus on your own well-being? Or do you feel guilty focusing on your own well-being?

    c. Do you believe taking care of self is actually unselfish, as you being whole and healthy is better positioned to care for others?

    d. What will you do by next Tuesday to improve your own well-being?

Chapter 29

The Visit

"Hi, Tom. Nice to see you again. So, you were recently in the emergency room. Tell me about that."

I couldn't believe it. Dr. Iuvenis had no idea why I was there.

"Doctor, didn't the hospital send over Tom's chart?"

God, I love you! I messaged telepathically to my bride.

"No. The only note I have is from your call the other day to book this appointment. Tom, why don't you just tell me why you were in the emergency room and how I can help you today?"

I was so glad Haylee was sitting next to me holding my hand. And so glad we had just spoken about the importance of love. Because even just sitting here, after being dropped off at the front door, waiting in line to check in, walking to the elevator, walking to the waiting room, sitting down, getting back up and walking to this exam room … I was exhausted. My chest was pounding. My head was pounding. And I was having trouble catching my breath.

Over the next seven minutes together, and as Dr. Iuvenis conducted a quick physical exam, we shared the 'Readers' Digest' version of my story and how I was feeling.

"So, what do we do now?"

Yes. I moved into solution mode.

"You should see a cardiologist for a work up. And with your symptoms of shortness of breath, feeling like you breathe better when sitting up, severe fatigue, chest pain and pressure, along with you mentioning your cardiac enzymes being elevated as well … yes, I think that would be the best next step."

"I know Dr. Schmidt at Cardiovascular Medical Group. He is contracted with our insurance. Would you please refer me to him?"

Dr. Schmidt was a good guy. He was also the lead doctor at C.M.G., and we had a relationship. If we were going down this pathway, he is who I wanted to see.

"Absolutely, Tom. I will have our referral specialist make the referral for you. Anything else I can do for you today?"

"No, I am good."

'Good?' Who was I kidding? Even Haylee knew I was scared.

REFLECTION

Serendipitously I received a number of blog posts, articles, studies, and stories with a similar relationship-centered theme.

Some examples:

– The blog post, "To connect with patients is key," by Dr. Craig Koniver

> *"If we are unable to connect with our patients, then it will not matter what prescriptions we write or supplements we recommend. Most of us pay this no attention. We go into the exam room and out again in a matter of minutes with prescriptions already printed."*

– The study, "Understanding Healing Relationships in Primary Care," from the Annals of Family Medicine

> *The purpose: "Clinicians often have an intuitive understanding of how their relationships with patients foster healing. Yet we know little empirically about the experience of healing and how it occurs between clinicians and patients. Our purpose was to create a model that identifies how healing relationships are developed and maintained. "*

> *The conclusion: "Healing relationships have an underlying structure and lead to important patient-centered outcomes."*

– An email from a dear friend and true leader working on the frontlines of the healthcare system

> *(Paraphrased) "Staff are not positioned to support the families in ways they should leading up to death. Families of dying loved ones are scared; they think that if they can just keep the person's heart beating, they won't have to feel the pain of loss. The nurses know what is coming, but the system fails the patients when nurses are not*

positioned to sit and share time with patients and/or families through the sadness of the dying process and talk with them about the fear and the unknown."

— *The blog post, "Compassionate care is a crucial component of care," by Joyce Hyam*

"We must reinforce the importance of providing compassionate care as it does make a positive impact on all of our lives."

These are all brilliant stories, so poignant, so impactful, so connected to the important things in healthcare ... and in life. And yet still to this day, these messages are not the norm when thinking about how to improve the healthcare system.

In fact, when was the last time you heard a healthcare leader say: "Let's improve the healthcare system by increasing the opportunities for healthcare providers (doctors, nurses, therapists, etc.) to truly connect with their patients"? Or "Let's invest in training our healthcare providers on how best to make an authentic connection, to establish relationship, to be emotionally intelligent, to be truly present, to listen, to engage, to empathize"?

Now think about this ...

10 percent of health outcomes is due to actual healthcare. The other 90 percent is due to health behaviors, socioeconomic factors, and the physical environment.

Digging into the numbers even deeper ... of the 10 percent of health outcomes due to healthcare, 90 percent of what physicians do involves connecting with patients and 10 percent involves the science, as taught in medical schools 30 years ago and highlighted in Dr. Craig Koniver's blog post.

Now taking this even further, based on these and other data, 1 percent of health outcomes is due to the science of medicine, 9 percent of health outcomes is due to practitioners connecting with their patients, 10 percent is due to the patients' physical environment, 40 percent is related to socioeconomic factors, and 40 percent comes from health behaviors.

If these data are correct (or even in the ballpark), it is even more imperative that healthcare system improvements (be they in care provision, delivery system changes, and/or reimbursement strategies) are in line with bringing relationship and connection back into the healing process. Technology, the latest pharmaceutical drug, a new surgical technique are all important to optimal healing. But they are not more important than the connection between a healthcare worker and a patient.

And if you don't believe me? Just look at the numbers.

Questions

1. As a healthcare leader, how are you ensuring physicians, nurses and other members of the care team are best positioned to achieve an optimal and authentic connection with their patients?

2. As a clinician, how are you ensuring that you and your patients are developing an authentic relationship and trust?

3. As a patient or family member, what (if any) do you see your role in developing an authentic connection with your clinician?

4. What barriers exist to ensuring that the 90 percent of the healthcare driver of health (the authentic connection) is maximized?

5. What are your recommendations to ensure these barriers are removed and healthcare provision is improved?

Chapter 30

Doctor's Orders

"Hi Tom. Nice to see you again. And this is?"

"This is my wife, Darlene."

"Hi, Darlene. I am Dr. Schmidt. I will be Tom's cardiologist."

I followed Dr. Schmidt down the long hallway toward the exam room. Neither of us saying a word. Me trying to keep my breaths under control knowing that my anxiety was only exacerbating my breathing difficulties.

Breathe, Tom. Breathe, was my first thought as we passed by a number of exam room doors, all closed.

Followed closely by, *I wish Doc was with me.*

By the time we entered the exam room I was exhausted, out of breath, and my chest was both heavy and painful.

"Have a seat in that chair, Tom."

Which I did with a louder grunt than I intended.

Hope he didn't notice that, went through my mind as Dr. Schmidt kept his eyes squarely on my chart.

"So, I have reviewed your test results from the hospital …"

"Oh, thank God," I thought. "My medical record got to him."

And then for the next twenty minutes or so, as Dr. Schmidt examined me, we discussed my history, my family history, my trip, how I felt then, how I felt upon my return, and how I was feeling now.

"Tell me about this elevated ANA. I see it marked both here at the time of your hospital stay as well as a notation in your history."

Now, of course, I do not have a clinical background, and at this point my mind was foggy at best. But I wanted to please and did my best to recall.

"I don't know about my ANA in the hospital," I began, "but rheumatoid arthritis runs in my family so I am a little familiar with the term."

"So tell me about your family's history of R.A."

Which I did to the best of my ability under the circumstances. *God, I wish Doc were here*, I thought again.

"And tell me more about your own ANA."

"When I was younger, soon after my bride and I were married…"

"Your bride? I like that. You still call your wife your bride. How long have you and Darlene been married?"

"Oh, we have been married nine years."

"Nine years. And still your bride? That is really sweet."

Although my head was now pounding too, this part of our discussion was almost enjoyable.

"Thank you. I believe I got it from my Dad. To this day he calls my Mom his bride. And they have been married about forty years."

"That is really wonderful. But go on. Sorry to derail you. You were saying when you were younger …"

"Yes, when I was younger I remember having an ANA test and then later getting a call to tell me to come right back into the office because my numbers were off the charts."

"And what happened then?"

"That is the funny (or sad) thing, Doctor. They scheduled me to come back in, which I did. Then they redid the test and then when those test results were received, they simply said, 'Well, the numbers are going down.' And that was it."

"Hmmmm …"

Of course, thinking back now, it made no since whatsoever to me that there was no follow up. I do recall my body being very inflamed and my joints aching, but then I always attributed that to my many injuries and surgeries.

"Anyway, it reminded me of the time I went to the hospital for a sprained ankle from basketball. After being treated I was sent home to where my Mémère must have been babysitting my sister. I remember limping in and Mémère saying to my parents, 'You need to take Tommy back to the hospital right now. They just called and said they found something else in his x-ray. They want you to go back'. Which we did. And when we did … nothing. We arrived at the hospital, and no one could tell us who called, why they called, or what we should do. So, we left again never receiving any additional information or follow through."

And then I added, "And no apology either."

"Hmmmm …" came the reply again. And then after a pause, "So were you ever diagnosed with an autoimmune disease like R.A.?"

"No."

"But you have had, on more than one occasion, elevated ANA test results, with at least one of those being extremely elevated. Correct?"

"That is right."

"And there is a history in the family."

"Yes."

"Okay."

"By the way, I don't know if this matters, but I have also had constant knee pain since I was very young."

I said this as I pictured one of those epic kickball games back in the day and then the pain that would follow as I limped home.

"I have seen many doctors, but no one has said conclusively what it is. And I have also had much pain in other joints over the years, but I just figure that is from my many sports injuries and subsequent surgeries."

Dr. Schmidt and I talked a bit more as we finished the physical exam and then he told me our game plan.

"Tom, first we are going to get a Holter monitor on you. We are also going to schedule you for another stress test. I also want you to see a rheumatologist and a neurologist. I want to rule out any autoimmune factors that may be in play here."

God, I wish Doc was here, I thought again as I tried to listen as my head and chest continued to pound.

"A what?"

"Don't worry. My staff will set you up with referrals and then you can be on your way. In the meantime, I want you resting."

"But when can I go back to work?"

"At this point, I want you to rest. Once I get all the results back, we will get you back in here. But for now, just rest."

"But …"

"No 'Buts.' Just rest."

Maybe it is a good thing Doc is not here, I thought. *Perhaps I don't have to tell her that I am supposed to just rest.*

"Tom, be patient. We will get the test results and then go from there. Any other questions?"

My mind was still foggy as I tried to process our discussion, *What is a Holter monitor and what does it do? Where do I get it? Why am I going to neurology? How do you know it is not the flu? Did Dr. Iuvenis's notes get to Dr. Schmidt? I need to get back to work. They are counting on me. What about my team? What about Mr. and Mrs. Jones? What about my family? What about my income? What about …*

But even though thoughts were flying around in my head all I replied was, "No. I am all set."

"Good. My nurse will be in to take care of you."

And then a few moments later …

"Tom, my name is Cindy. Okay, Dr. Schmidt has lots of orders for you. Why don't you follow me to the front desk? There we can make sure we get all of these taken care of."

Orders? I thought. *I am being ordered to rest? I am being ordered to get a monitor? I am being ordered to see other doctors? And who are they, and how do I know if they are any good? Orders? There has got to be a better way.*

REFLECTION

Being the dad of Miss Maine USA 2014 still feels brand new, even as my daughter Samantha over the past many years continues to leverage this experience as part of her life journey.

During her reign, Sammy had amazing opportunities to support such worthy causes as the Muscular Dystrophy Association, Camp Sunshine, Maine Women's Fund, and so many others as she learned, grew, and blossomed.

During this time, she also opted to create and follow a course that leads to the modeling industry. And with my mind always processing, this is where I rediscovered the importance of Swanson's Caring Model to achieving optimal outcomes.

The model:

- *Knowing the patient (seeing the world through their eyes)*
- *Being with the patient (and building trust)*
- *Doing for the patient (being appropriately of service balanced with ...)*
- *Empowering the patient (teaching, coaching, explaining)*
- *Maintaining belief (having faith in and esteem for the patient)*

As my three children have grown, I have been blessed to have a schedule that allowed me to be with them and see their world through their eyes. To see the paths they chose, the challenges they faced, and the desire, passion and light that shines when they are on their path. To see them achieve and fail, learn and grow and get stronger, and to identify ways with them in which I can most be helpful as they also establish their own footing.

So in the Fall of 2015, when my daughter told my wife and me that she was scheduled to go to modeling school as she continued on a new path birthed through her hard work and her reign as Miss Maine USA, and with Kristen Swanson's care model in mind, I pondered:

- *How does a dad see this new world (of modeling) through his daughter's eyes?*

- *How does a dad be with his daughter in this new world?*

And then answered: "This dad goes to modeling school!"

Now, one might think that an almost fifty-year-old healthcare executive doesn't belong in modeling school. And yet, there I was. And it was an amazing experience.

Sammy and I learned which colors to wear for "go-sees," tax implications of modeling in multiple states, how to "slate," and which states to focus significant energy and attention on and which not — together. I saw Sammy in her element, and I got to know my daughter in a far more complete way as I was seeing her world through her eyes.

So why do I share this story?

Ensuring time, relationship, and trust at each and every healing encounter is essential to optimal care and outcomes and allows for truly listening to the patient's whole story; both knowing the patient and being with the patient (to use Kristen Swanson's words); the co-creation of care paths, and the impact of doing so…

- *Improved patient and physician engagement*
- *Better adherence to the co-created care plans*
- *Improved patient safety*
- *Improved outcomes, e.g., patient's emotional health, symptoms, pain levels*

… and thus better care … healthCARING.

My daughter telling me about her experience in less than 10 minutes with me interrupting within the first 23 seconds would not have allowed for optimal communication and would only provide part of the full picture. It would only provide me with a tidbit of an amazing and educational story which I would then try to use to inform decision-making. Less than ideal for sure and yet that is our current healthcare model.

Sammy's modeling career is very important to her and my role as a father necessitated me following the path above so that I was best positioned to support and honor Sammy as she continues on her journey.

As healthcare leaders (models or not), we must also create paths (care models) which allow clinicians to be with and know their patients through their patients' eyes if we truly want to improve care provision. If we don't ... we will miss out on something special ... as I would have with Sammy.

Questions

1. As a clinician, how important is it for a patient and family to understand doctor's orders?

    a. Why is the term "orders" used?

    b. When, if at all, should a care plan be co-created between a patient and family and their doctor?

2. As a clinician, patient or family member, when should a care plan be dictated by the doctor?

Chapter 31

The Robot

"Okay kids, we need to drive Daddy into Portland to see the doctor. Get ready."

"Daddy needs to see another doctor? Why does he have so many doctors?"

"They just want to be sure Daddy is getting better, so they are being very careful, Sam. Don't you worry."

"Do you think Daddy is getting better, Momma?"

I wish I could have seen Doc's face as she was having this discussion with Sammy. Or perhaps maybe it was better that I could not. They were near the door to the garage getting shoes on as I was still sitting on the couch waiting until the last second to stand and walk to the van. Only faintly could I hear …

"Yes, Sammy. Daddy is getting stronger each day. Now please go get Haylee and Tommy while I make sure your father is ready to go."

Eventually we were all loaded into the van, with me shunning Doc's assistance. (Honestly, I was tired of being reliant on others. I would rather fall on my face than continue to be a burden.)

This day my chest pain was less intense, but my breathing was harder and my head continued to pound even with the daily Vioxx.

"We almost there, Doc?"

"I think so. The building should be up around the corner on Washington Street somewhere."

The folks from Dr. Schmidt's office had provided us with a referral and directions for me to be equipped with the Holter monitor.

I learned from Doc that this device will monitor my heart for 24 continuous hours and, in this case, the readings will be recorded remotely. My understanding was that it will help Dr. Schmidt correlate my symptoms, such as my chest pain, with rhythm changes that may be signs of ischemia or reduced blood supply to my heart.

"Doc, this time I would like to go in to the appointment alone."

Perhaps because the thought of me continuing to burden those I love most was exacerbated or perhaps something else. All I knew at this time was I needed to be alone (or at least alone at this next visit).

"Tom? Why? The kids will be fine. We can all go in. What is the matter?"

"Oh it is not that, Doc. I think this time it would just be best. And hey, there is a McDonald's nearby. Why don't you take the kids to 'D-Donalds'," which is what Haylee calls it, "while I get the monitor and we will meet when I am done."

After a little more discussion, Doc finally agreed to let me go it alone. I felt bad that I may have hurt her feelings, and I knew that I will process that for a long time, but I also knew for some reason I needed to 'walk on my own two feet' again. Which may not sound like much seeing that I was simply walking from the van to a doctor's office, but for me at this moment, it meant a great deal.

As Doc drove off, very slowly I noticed, I turned and faced the building. It was all red brick. Probably built in the 80's. Two stories tall with lots of blacked out glass.

Luckily for me my appointment was on the first floor.

"Hi, I am Tom Dahlborg, and I am here to get a Holter monitor."

"Oh yes, Mr. Dahlborg. Dr. Schmidt's office called. Just have a seat, and we will be with you momentarily. In the meantime, please fill out the forms on this clipboard and when done return to me. Oh yeah, do you also have your insurance card?"

I sat down with my head pounding and began to try to remember how many knee surgeries I had had and when they all were, along with the lymph node removal from my neck, surgery on my back to remove some sort of mass, and so on and so on, so that I could complete the many pages of paperwork before me.

Allergies to medications? Well, after one knee surgery the Vicodin they prescribed made me itchy, I thought as I made note of Vicodin as an allergen.

My maternal grandparents' medical history? My paternal grandparents' medical history? My God, my head hurts! I thought.

"Mr. Dahlborg, my name is Carol. I will take you back now."

Carol greeted me from a doorway across the waiting room. Dressed in what I would call business casual clothing, she had short brown hair and a kind smile.

"How are you today?"

Hmmmm … I actually had no idea how to answer her question, I realized. *Is this a standard 'how are you?' or is she really asking as if the answer will impact my visit today?*

"I am okay. How are you?"

"I am very well, Thomas."

"Tom is fine."

"Well then I am very well, Tom. Now come right in here and have a seat in the green chair."

As I looked into the exam room, I noticed two chairs. One appeared to be yellow, so the other I was hoping was green. I slowly made my way to it and sat down.

"So I am going to set you up with your Holter monitor today. Do you understand why you are having this done?"

"I believe so."

"Well, good, but just in case let me explain a bit more," which Carol did as I tried to regain my breath from the walk down the hallway.

"Any questions?"

"I don't think so."

Even if I did, with my head pounding as it was, I don't believe I would have retained the answers. Just as I didn't really retain her description of the Holter monitor.

Perhaps I should have had Doc join me? I thought, but then again knew Doc could and would explain more when we got home if need be. "

"Okay, remove your shirt so we can attach the electrodes."

As I did, I made note of how tight my shoulders, traps, and neck were. *No wonder I have another headache,* I thought.

"You have quite the hairy chest, we will have to do a bit of landscaping," Carol said with a smile as she turned to get a plastic razor.

"Okay, a little clearing here and here and here. And now a bit of alcohol to ensure good attachments, and we will be in good shape."

Carol attached the electrodes, I believe there were five, and then handed me the monitor.

"This is the Holter monitor unit itself. And with these attachments we will be monitoring your EKG remotely for the next 24 hours. The unit is fairly large and you have a number of wires attached so you will want to be very mindful of your movements."

Already I could feel the attachments pulling at the remaining hair on my chest.

"Let's place this strap around your neck and also clip the unit to your waist band. That way it will be well secured."

Around my neck? Ugh.

But rather than speak up I simply followed orders. Looking back, I think Doc would have asked for other options for me.

"There. Now let's put your jersey back on over the unit and see how that feels."

Very slowly but surely, Carol and I pulled my t-shirt over my head and then placed my hands and arms through the arm holes as we further pulled the jersey down over the electrodes, wires, and monitor unit.

"There you go. How does that feel?"

"It feels fine. Thank you, Carol." I managed to say as the pressure in my chest began to build again and my dry cough could not continue to be withheld.

Cough Cough Cough

"Well, then. You are good to go. Do you have a ride?"

"I do. My wife and kids should be back from getting D-Donald's. Um … I mean, McDonald's. D-Donald's is what my youngest calls it," I quickly explained.

"Mmmmm … A Big Mac and Fries does sound good right about now. Perhaps that will be my lunch," Carol replied as we both laughed at the irony of the need for Holter monitors and McDonald's.

Squinting as I walked out of the office door, I could barely see our van parked directly across from me.

"Daddy!" I heard coming my way as the rays of the sun continued to shine on me.

"Sammy!" I remember calling back as I thought about her beautiful smile awaiting me.

As I got a bit closer, I no longer heard the giggles and laughter of my children but rather Tommy squeal, "Daddy! You look like one of my robots!"

"Yeah, Dad. You look like a robot!" Sammy added quickly.

As I reached the side of the van, I could now see my three beautiful children looking at me ... but a bit *creeped out* as they would say.

"Wow, Tom. Pull up your shirt."

"Okay, Doc," I replied as I slowly lifted the waist of my t-shirt up toward my chest.

"That monitor is huge. I didn't think the unit would be that big."

I, of course, had no expectation.

"Daddy, Tommy and Sammy are right. You look like a robot. And I don't like it," added Haylee.

As I slowly stepped a bit closer to the van and its open back window so the kids could see me better I responded, "This thing you see is going to help me heal. It is going to help me feel better." And then added, "It is just like a radio. And it is going to send information, like we get when we listen to the radio, to my doctor."

"Wow. That is cool, Dad."

Phew.

"Thanks, Tommy. And you know what?"

"What, Dad?"

"Even if I was a robot ..."

Okay, admittedly I was taking a risk here.

"... this robot has a heart that loves you three very, very much. In fact, aside from Momma, the biggest heart ever because it is full of so much love for you."

"I love you too, Dad. But a Dad-Robot would be wicked cool, too!"

REFLECTION

There is a very important place for technology in the future of healthcare... when incorporated mindfully.

When technology becomes the be-all and end-all 'solution,' doctors and nurses and patients and families get lost and great harm is likely.

When technology is incorporated as part of a co-created care path and with the intention to enhance the healing journey and improve the connection between patients, families and clinicians, then each stakeholder will be honored and whole, and the technological tool will be achieving its true raison d'etre.

Questions

1. As a healthcare leader, clinician, staff person, patient or family member, how do you see technology transforming healthcare in the future?

    a. Where do you see this transformation improving care?

    b. Where do you see this transformation worsening care?

    c. What do you foresee as the unintended consequences (both positive and negative) of the technological transformation of healthcare?

2. As a healthcare leader, how would you fan or mitigate the unintended consequence?

3. How do you explain complex and perhaps scary concepts to young children?

Chapter 32

The Call

"Mrs. Dahlborg. Is your husband okay?"

I was not the best patient by any means. And by me not wanting to burden my bride with every ache and pain, I surely was not good at keeping her abreast of my condition.

"Is my husband okay? Who is this?"

"This is Laura. We provided Tom with the Holter monitor."

"I don't understand."

"Mrs. Dahlborg. We are monitoring Tom's EKG remotely. His graph is off the chart. I am calling to check in and to ensure he is getting the medical assistance he needs."

Unbeknownst to Doc, I had been in extreme discomfort since our outing to get the monitor. Be it over exertion or what I didn't know. Of course, I told myself that "this flu is really kicking my butt."

My chest pain had increased to the point where the only way I could describe it was crushing. My breathing was worse and my cough worsening.

I, of course, didn't know she was on the phone with the Holter monitor folks.

"Tom! Tom! Are you okay?"

"Am I okay?" I thought. That is a strange question seeing that we have been living this together for a very long time.

"Yes Doc," *Cough Cough*, "I am okay. Same as usual."

"No sense in stressing Doc out," I figured.

"He says he is about the same."

"Mrs. Dahlborg, please keep an eye on him and call 911 if things worsen. Dr. Schmidt will be getting the results shortly."

Doc hung up and then headed into the living room where I was planted in my usual spot on the couch with Angus on my lap.

"Tom, I just got the strangest call."

REFLECTION

For a number of years, I had the privilege of coaching a group of high school basketball players.

It was during this time that I was traveling for business and had to miss a game and asked my assistant coach to lead the team. And as I was enjoying a quiet dinner a few states away I received the following text:

"Halftime. Us 19 them 20. Timmy mad."

Once I realized the text came from my assistant coach's wife and that she would communicate with her husband, I responded:

"Tell Timmy he will shoot better when he is relaxed. Also tell him to use his aggression under the boards."

I soon inquired about the other team's defense and called an offensive play.

"Basket."

We continued our texting, and I learned of a defensive lapse. No problem. It was corrected with a little encouragement from afar.

More information was shared, and I found myself truly engaged in the game and cheering the team on from hundreds of miles away.

Question about an offensive set. No problem. Text.

Team down a bit emotionally. No problem. Text.

And eventually I learned through the wonders of technology that we had won a hard-fought game.

But was that the best text I received that night? No. The best text I received actually came after the game and simply said: "Boys loved hearing from you!"

Over the next few days, I thought about the lessons that could be extrapolated from this experience and applied to the use of technology in healthcare. And in doing so I realized the authentic connection among my players, assistant coach and I created the climate that allowed for this successful use of technology.

The climate we created included:

Time – Sharing hundreds of hours together on and off the court

Continuity – Coaching with my assistant for eight years and together coaching eight of our eleven players over multiple years.

Mindfulness – Remaining in relationship to what we are going through at any given time, holding it, honoring it, and befriending it and one another

Presence – Preserving a non-judgmental receptivity to the experience of players, coaches and families alike as on and off court challenges have arisen

Humility – An absolute willingness to abandon preconceived suppositions if information (be it verbal or non-verbal) from a player, family or coach is not in alignment

Empathy – Maintaining an intention to recognize and honor emotions that are being experienced by my players, families and assistant coach

Authentic Relationship – The culmination of all the above in trust, reliance, safety, and belief in one another, our team and our community

Also, through this experience I recognized that without this climate, there would not have been an openness to text me initially; I would not have known what was needed and when, or when not, to intervene. The players would not have adhered to my instruction from afar, my assistant coach would not have been open to additional insights, and if I did insert myself through the use of technology, I could have done harm.

Technology should neither be demonized nor held as the one and only solution to our healthcare challenges. Rather, technology should be leveraged to supplement healing encounters and optimize health outcomes, and courageous adaptive leaders must guard it from being used for any contrary purpose.

Questions

1. As a patient, how often are you fully open with what you are experiencing health wise? If not 100%, why?

2. As a clinician, how important is it that you know what the person in your care is experiencing?

    a. How do you ensure open communication?

    b. How are you leveraging technology to enhance care without losing the humanity of caring?

Chapter 33

The Heart Attack

After ensuring Tommy and Sammy were off to school, and Haylee was safely in the hands of our closer than ever friend Hope, Doc and I had made our way to the next doctor's office for my stress test.

The first and last stress test I had had was the day after my trip to the ER. I was clearly in a lot more dis-stress at that time. And yet on this day, I felt my innards shaking as thoughts and potential new realities crossed my mind.

'What if's' were entering my thought processes more and more each day. 'What if I am really sick?' 'What if I don't improve?' 'What if I die?'

That last thought I usually dispelled quite quickly and yet today…

"Doc," I began to say as she drove us north on Route One again toward the southern Maine mecca of medical care.

But as I did, I could see she was biting the side of her mouth again.

I almost shared how scared I was. I almost shared how much discomfort I was in. I almost shared how much I didn't want anything to happen to me while I am undergoing this test.

But I thought the better of it as I saw the sparkle of her blue eyes even more so this morning.

Instead I reached over and took her hand in mine and said, "I am so sorry for all of this. You are doing so much for me."

As Doc turned to me while also maintaining focus on the road, I continued, "Once I pass this test and get the green light from Dr. Schmidt, I promise to take better care of myself. I promise."

"Oh Tom, we both know how you are wired," began her reply. Then, "Now clearly your mother didn't tell me everything about you and how your mind works prior to us getting married and committing to 'in sickness and in health', so I do have a bone to pick with her…"

I began to smile as this had been our running joke since my first health issue just after our wedding, which led to an Arubian honeymoon visit to the ER.

"… but after nine years I now know you quite well, so while your promises are appreciated, I will not be holding my breath."

With this we both broke into laughter … at least until my coughing fit forced me to stop.

Cough Cough Cough

"I do so love you, Doc."

"And I love you too, or I would have left you at the ER after you ruined Tommy's first birthday."

Doc was on a roll.

I then decided to continue to avoid acknowledging my fear by discussing process and process improvement opportunities to both keep my mind busy but also with the thought that when I get the clearance I could leverage this information at work.

"Can you tell me again how many calls it took to make this appointment and about the confusion?"

Doc looked at me like I had three heads … but then responded. I believe she too realized this discussion could also serve to take her mind off of what we really should be discussing.

"At first, Dr. Schmidt's office was going to schedule this appointment. But when we did not hear by the next day from them, I called. They then said that your primary care doctor needed to schedule it and prior approval would need to be granted by our insurance company. So, I then called Dr. Iuvenis's office."

I could see Doc getting 'ticked off,' as my father would say, as she continued.

"And when I did, it took forever to get hold of live person. But when I did, they said they had not received any orders or information of any kind from Dr. Schmidt's office and thus they could not do anything. They in turn suggested I call his office again and ask them to send over the information."

Oh yes, Doc was now getting animated. "God, I was glad she could multitask so well," I thought as she navigated traffic and continued.

"So I called Dr. Schmidt's office again. They told me everything had been sent. Well, at this point that wasn't good enough, so I told them to resend it and to let me know when it is done. And that they needed to do so immediately."

I love when she gets tough.

"They then told me they will fax it over immediately and that I can call them back if there are still questions. I gave it thirty minutes and then called your primary's office again who still said they didn't receive it. I then called Dr. Schmidt's office back and again had to wait to get someone else on the line."

Doc was no longer biting the side of her mouth … but she was turning quite red.

"Well, that person told me that in fact your primary does NOT need to make the referral but rather Dr. Schmidt's office should. That we actually did not need to go back to our PCP. 'Well, that is great! Thanks for the runaround', I thought. But then I said, 'wait a minute', that is great regarding the referral, but my husband's PCP still needs to know what is going on. How will that information be sent to him?'"

God, I love her! I remember thinking.

"'Oh, don't worry.' They told me. 'But I am worrying. This is ridiculous.' I wanted to say. But decided at this point to let that go and focus on the referral and this test."

Doc then continued …

"They stressed me out and confused me. And I am a nurse and have worked in the system for a long time."

I made a mental note of all of these access and care barriers.

"That is so insane, Doc." I said prior to continuing with another coughing fit.

Cough Cough Cough

And with each cough, I promised myself that I would get back to work and with my team fix this and other brokenness within our system for our patients. For Mr. and Mrs. Jones.

Once we arrived at the office Doc parked the minivan and then came around and met me as I walked toward the front of it. From there together, arm-in-arm, we walked toward the front door (albeit slowly). Each leaning on each other. Me with my chest pained. Doc with her heart pained.

"I am going to be alright," I tried to say but with my cough only get out, "I am goi…."

"Shhhhhhh. We are almost there. Save your strength for kicking ass on the test."

"Hi, I am Tom Dahlborg. I am here for a stress test."

"Who?"

"Tom Dahlborg. Dr. Schmidt referred me."

"Wait a minute. Can you spell that for me?"

"Sure, D-A-H-L-B- …"

"Oh wait. I got you. You are one of the heart attacks."

REFLECTION

More and more, we read that hospital nurses suffer from depression at twice the average rate.

And the problem isn't confined to the United States.

Amid government calls to reduce patient wait times for beds, a nurse in London was working in a closed hospital ward where the Pseudomembranous colitis (PMC) virus was running rampant.

After a death on the ward "opened up" a bed, hospital leadership ordered the bed be filled. This nurse informed me that leadership made it very clear, "The government had set a wait time standard, and they were going to achieve it. No matter what."

The hospital leaders ignored the nurse's protests and admitted a sick elderly woman to the closed ward.

"She contracted PMC and shortly thereafter died," the nurse said.

This encounter impacted this nurse profoundly. The patient's unnecessary death. The total disregard for the wisdom of those on the front lines by leadership. The clear disrespect for nursing.

Yes, each component of this story harmed this nurse. There are significant adverse effects on clinical quality, patient experience and safety, as well as staff satisfaction and retention when the folks on the frontlines, i.e., nurses, medical assistants, front desk staff, are not listened to and not honored.

Many times, what we experience in healthcare, now referred to as patient experience, is a reflection of the experience and the treatment of well-meaning staff.

The healthcare system is a complex adaptive system ... and only when we see it as such and stop mistreating healthcare staff, while expecting these same folks to provide empathetic, compassionate, safe and effective healthcare will we truly improve the system for all those we care about.

Questions

1. As a clinician, have you ever referred to a patient by their diagnosis?

    a. Is it important to see a patient with a diagnosis as a whole person? If so, why? If not, why not?

    b. Does seeing a patient as primarily a diagnosis improve care, outcomes and safety or not? How do you know?

2. As a patient, have you ever been referred to as a diagnosis and if so, how did that make you feel?

3. As a healthcare leader, are you truly listening to your staff? If so, how does this manifest?

4. As a staff person, are you mistreated?

    a. Are you burning out?

    b. Or do you feel valued?

    c. Do you have support?

    d. Are you listened to?

    e. Are you appreciated?

    f. How do you know?

Chapter 34

Lose Me Forever

Thirty minutes later, and after I had completed a new set of forms I heard, "Mr. Dahlborg, my name is Michelle, and I will be helping you with your stress test today."

For some reason I did not look back to see Doc as I followed Michelle. I think perhaps I didn't want to say goodbye.

"Tom, have you had a stress test before?"

"Oh yes. The day after my admission to the hospital."

"Okay. Then this will be old news to you."

I don't think so.

After we were in the room and I stripped down to my shorts, Michelle began to place the electrodes on my chest.

"You may feel a slight burning or stinging sensation."

I did for sure. But worse was the pulling of my chest hair as the electrodes were positioned and then repositioned.

Note to self, shave chest prior to any more stress tests, I thought as I also thought about what a difference could be made if in fact the nurse or technician or somebody would have simply shaved my entire chest, or just the spots for the electrodes, or even let me know ahead of time to do so myself if I so chose. Clearly this wasn't number one on my mind as a I was scheduled for the test and yet now, I was thinking about how these electrodes were going to be pulled off once the test was completed and how each one would be pulling my chest hair out by their roots. "Ouch."

Such a little thing and yet also such a little thing to improve the experience of a patient.

Yes, note to self to bring back to work. What other 'little things' that are actually quite important for patients and families are we missing?

Once the electrodes were all set and the blood pressure cuff around my arm, again not the extra-large one even though I requested, I was led to the treadmill and positioned for the test to begin.

She is very nice, I remember thinking, *but Michelle is not hearing me. Being nice is important. But so is truly listening with the intent to understand.*

"Okay, Tom. We will take baseline readings of your blood pressure and heart rate. From there you will feel the blood pressure cuff inflate every few minutes. It may feel tight …"

It already does.

"… Okay. You can begin walking now."

And as I had done so the morning after my hospital admission, I began to walk. And as I did, and as the pace and incline increased, I began to experience a shortness of breath and more discomfort in my chest and then a coughing fit which almost knocked me off of the machine.

"Tom? Are you okay?"

"I am fine," I remember stammering. And then trying to make light of it, "If I fell all the way off, we could have won $10,000 on America's Funniest Videos."

We both laughed hesitantly as I regained my footing, and then shortly thereafter, although it felt like hours, I finished the test.

"Mrs. Dahlborg, Tom did fine."

I didn't hear what or if Doc asked anything but was pleased to hear, "I did fine".

"Great. What happens next?"

"We will send the results to Tom's cardiologist. Dr. Schmidt, right? And he will be in touch with you directly regarding next steps. Do you have any questions?"

"Will Dr. Iuvenis, Tom's PCP, also get the results?"

"He should, as long as we have his information in our system. Which again, we should," responded Michelle.

I am not sure if Doc believed her or not, but I was tired and after looking into my eyes, Doc realized I needed to get home.

"Doc, please just take me home or lose me forever."

Like I have always said, "Nothing like a pseudo-Top Gun movie quote after a stress test."

REFLECTION

"During the Korean War, the Navy kill ratio was twelve-to-one. We shot down twelve of their jets for every one of ours. In Vietnam, this ratio fell to three-to-one. Our pilots depended on missiles. They lost their 'dog-fighting' skills."

~ Jester, Top Gun, 1986

I remember seeing the movie Top Gun in the mid-1980s and how this quote struck me ... and believe it or not ... it has informed much of my work in healthcare.

Fifty plus years ago (1964) the Hippocratic Oath was rewritten by Louis Lasagna, Academic Dean of the School of Medicine at Tufts University, to include (excerpts):

- *I will apply, for the benefit of the sick, all measures [that] are required, avoiding those twin traps of overtreatment and therapeutic nihilism.*

- *I will remember that there is art to medicine as well as science, and that warmth, sympathy, and understanding may outweigh the surgeon's knife or the chemist's drug.*

- *I will remember that I do not treat a fever chart, a cancerous growth, but a sick human being, whose illness may affect the person's family and economic stability.*

- *... may I long experience the joy of healing those who seek my help.*

Thirty years ago, medical schools taught that the most important component of a mental health healing encounter is empathy, human connection, and authentic relationship between a physician and patient.

And yet more recently we healthcare leaders have evolved the healthcare delivery system to include:

- *Clinicians triple booked every 15 minutes*

- *8- to 12-minute office visits*

- *The I-Patient (to borrow from Dr. Abraham Verghese) replacing the actual patient*

- *Patients being dehumanized and becoming a diagnosis rather than a whole person*

- *Clinician focus turning away from the human being before them and toward electronic health records, target organs and test results*

- *Technology becoming the solution focus rather than a tool*

- *Care teams held to the same productivity standards as clinicians (as noted above), yet providing less continuity for a patient with "their" clinician*

- *A model that rewards excessive tests and invasive procedures*

- *Physicians and nurses burning out and worse*

We have switched from "dog fighting," i.e., avoiding overtreatment, establishing and ensuring human connection and authentic relationship, and finding joy in healing to "missile dependency," i.e., the "evolved" model described above.

In our effort to make things better, we have forgotten why we are here in the first place. We have sought "missiles" to improve the broken system. We have lost our way. And we are harming those we should be honored to serve.

If we truly want to improve the health of our patients, families, and communities, it is time to break our addiction to missiles and reconnect with the Hippocratic Oath, what was taught in medical schools thirty years ago, and most importantly to our patients, families, and communities.

For only then will we truly innovate healthcare.

Questions

1. As a clinician, how has technology improved the care you provide? How has technology hindered your ability to provide good care? Please share stories.

2. As a patient, please share stories of the use of technology and its impact (positive or negative) on your or a loved one's health and healing?

3. What recommendations would you make to ensure technology is leveraged appropriately in order to optimize care?

Chapter 35

Setting Records

Dr. Schmidt was very clear. He developed a plan for me, and I was following it to a 'T', as my father would say.

Next step: Neurology.

"All signs and symptoms are pointing to cardiac. I cannot help you."

Well, good. I would not want to be treated by him anyway.

Yes, my medical record did not arrive at the neurologist's office in time.

Note to self, for now on carry my own medical record with me.

And, yes, the neurologist seemed very busy.

But can a specialist, even the best of the best, truly determine that he or she cannot help a patient without a physical exam, with only a cursory glance away from the computer, and in less than 7 minutes?

So yes, the reaction I shared with Doc when we were both safely back in our minivan was a mix of disappointment and dismay.

Next step: Rheumatology.

"Yes, I see you have had elevated ANAs in the past. And yes, I understand that your family has a history of Rheumatoid Arthritis …"

I was so glad I carried my own chart to this appointment.

"… but all indications point to a cardiac event. I cannot help you."

Back in the minivan …

"But Doc, I thought it was important to understand the root cause of the cardiac event?"

"It is, Tom. It is."

Next step: Pulmonology.

"I don't see any indication of a PE. I cannot help you."

"Three appointments over three weeks and a total of seventeen minutes." We were setting records. (Or were we? Is it like this for everyone?) "Who's next?"

REFLECTION

Years later I was leading what would now be called an "innovation laboratory." During this time, we were integrating medical and behavioral health, addressing health equity with new concepts and models, revolutionizing healthcare leadership, and developing a care model that served to heal the clinician as much as the patient and family. And it was during this time, as part of our research, I heard stories from many physicians and nurses alike about how they were burning out in the traditional medical model. They shared how they felt like cogs in a machine making widgets rather than as healers caring for their patients. They told of how they 'lost their soul for healing,' and how this translated into unhealthy behaviors leading to harm of self and of others.

And it was these stories and many others, and these clinicians (many who opted to become disruptive innovators themselves), that helped to inform, provide a different lens, and position me to see the challenges that I felt as a patient from a whole new perspective. The perspective of a broken system where many of us have contributed to creating it and only together would we be able to fix it.

Questions

1. As a healthcare leader, clinician, staff person, patient, or family member, what are the flames of goodness within the healthcare system that we must fan?

    a. What are the top areas of the healthcare system where fixes are required?

    b. What recommendations would you make to ensure we are fanning the flames of goodness and fixing the brokenness?

    c. How would you ensure the people within the system; i.e., the doctors and nurses, patients and families, and all who engage with the healthcare system, are best positioned to honor themselves and their callings and be of service to others?

Chapter 36

Blanket of Red

"Doc, are you ready for this? Today is the day!"

I actually slept the previous night. I am not sure why. Perhaps simply out of exhaustion or perhaps knowing that this was the day I got my test results.

"Today we finally hear that I have," dramatic pause for affect, "the flu!"

"You know you are killing me, don't you?"

"I know. It is why you love me, right?"

"Not so much, Tom. Not so much."

As we rode to Dr. Schmidt's office, I remember thinking about the emotional toll a patient and family experiences when facing a (in my case at this point) potentially serious diagnosis and how this toll may manifest.

I wondered if my organization's doctors and nurses, front desk staff, receptionists, claims reviewers, well actually everyone on my team … if we were all aware? I wondered if we were able to truly put ourselves in another's place when the wife of a patient requests a coated tablet for her husband. I wondered if we could truly empathize and then put that empathy into action with the husband who was 'losing it' at the reception desk after he has learned his wife has cancer. I wondered if we truly understood what was going on for people prior to judging them as disruptive or worse.

I continued to process these thoughts for a couple of reasons. The first being it took my mind off of my situation and the stress it was placing on my own family, and second because I was feeling more and more guilty every day that I was not with my team honoring my commitment to them and to Mrs. Jones to help make things better.

As the ride continued so did my processing, *And what about my team? What if Cathy learned her child was seriously ill? Or Frank's wife?* Had I positioned my team to care for one another in both thought and in action? Prior to my becoming ill, would I as a leader have known what to do? Did I now? Did I foster the types of relationships where we could share these feelings? Share our whole selves? Had I dropped the proverbial ball when it came to creating a safe place and a safe space for this type of sharing? I had put so much pressure on my team to achieve our aim in such a short timeframe … was my focus and my approach actually detrimental to both my team and our goal achievement?

"Doc, I need to get back to work."

"Tom, nice to see you again. And hello, Darlene. Both of you come on in."

Yes, Doc was joining me!

"Well, Tom, here is where we are, I have received your Holter monitor and your stress test results. Now you also saw a neurologist too, correct?"

"Yes."

"Excellent. But wait I do not have his notes yet. I will be right back."

As Dr. Schmidt left, I could feel my hands begin to shake as the blood left my face. *Hide your hands, Tom,* I said to myself.

Okay, I told myself, *focus outside of me. Focus away from me.*

"You okay, Doc? He will be right back. I bet he is having the notes faxed to him."

"Oh yes, Tom. I am fine. Watching my husband …," Doc's voice trailed off as I could see her blue eyes puddle once again.

"I am going to be fine. I promise."

Looking deeply into my bride's eyes, I could see how her still beautiful blue eyes which once shined on a bed of snow now glistened on a blanket of red. And as I gazed, I could only imagine how I would feel if our roles were reversed, the stress, the worry, the games my mind would play, and the exhaustion.

We held each other's gaze for an eternity before Doc blinked a few times, wiped her eyes and then placed her hands on my knee and said, "I know, Tom. I know."

About fifteen minutes later, Dr. Schmidt returned to our exam room with a fax in his hands.

"Okay, now we have the stress test, Holter monitor and notes from neurology, rheumatology, and pulmonology."

I believe I had seen one or two more –ologies but for the life of me I could not remember.

"Okay, this is what we have so far. All your symptoms, all the test results … By the way, what happened with the Holter monitor?"

"What do you mean?"

"Your graph was off the chart. I see a notation that you were contacted. What had happened? What were you experiencing?"

This is one of those times I wish Doc was not in the room with me. Clearly an issue I needed to get over. I didn't want to alarm her. I didn't want her to stress more.

"I think I was just experiencing some discomfort," I replied with as much sincerity as I could muster as I also thought about other patient's and whether they disclose as much as they should.

Another challenge to undertake when I am back to work.

"Hmmmm … must have been a great deal of discomfort."

Don't look at Doc. Don't look at Doc. Just play it cool.

"Well," Dr. Schmidt began again, "this is where we are. All your symptoms, all you are experiencing, all your test results to date, and the other specialist's findings all point to a cardiac event. And at this time, Tom and Darlene, I believe we are going to find that you have …"

Of course, I was still holding out hope that 'the flu' were to be the next two words uttered.

"… what is known as viral myocarditis."

"Viral myo…," was all I could catch as my mind tried to engulf what I heard.

"Myocarditis is a disease marked by inflammation and damage of the heart muscle. It usually attacks otherwise healthy people and can have many causes. It is believed that 5 to 20% of all cases of sudden death in young adults are due to myocarditis," Dr. Schmidt explained.

Wow, I really didn't need to know that stat, I thought. *And neither did Doc.*

Dr. Schmidt continued, "There are many causes of myocarditis, including viral infections, thus the 'viral' aspect of this myocarditis. But it can also be caused by autoimmune diseases. With your story of a plane flight, sudden onset, illness, they all point us to viral myocarditis. And yet, you have a family history of rheumatoid arthritis, you have had significantly elevated ANA's and considerable joint pain, so I am still open that perhaps this was caused by an autoimmune disease. But for now, our working diagnosis is 'viral myocarditis.'"

Of course my mind went to, *Whoa ... whoa ... this is not right. I am thirty-five years old. I have been a pseudo-athlete all of my life. I did not have a 'cardiac-event'. No way!*

"Doctor, so what does this mean? What is our next step?"

"Darlene, I want Tom to undergo a cardiac catheterization procedure. This way we will be able to assess both deterioration of the heart muscle and/or inflammation."

"What are the risks?"

"We do these all the time, Darlene. But yes, in rare circumstances, there are risks such as blood clots, collapsed lung, injury to the artery, and such, but again only on rare occasions."

"Doctor, how does this procedure help my recovery?"

"Tom, the procedure will help to confirm our diagnosis."

Dr. Schmidt's response made great sense to me at the time. Once we knew exactly what was going on, then we would be able to treat it. And knowing myself, with clarity comes focus and no matter what, I knew I would do everything in my power to get healthy again.

"Who schedules the cardiac cath, and where is it done?"

"My office will take care of all the scheduling, Tom. We will do the procedure at Maine Med. We will get this scheduled ASAP."

I remember being afraid to look at Doc. Now not only has it been confirmed that I had a 'cardiac event,' but now I would be having an invasive procedure. More stress on my love. *But clearly must be done, right?*

But I did. I did look over at my bride and as each tear rolled down her cheek, I realized that the sadness I was causing her broke my heart more than any virus ever could.

REFLECTION

I remember one day perusing the USA TODAY when a particular headline in the Sports Section grabbed my attention:

"NASCAR needs its own team of traveling doctors"

And then reading within the article:

> *"But he never got a chance to race because NASCAR parked him for medical reasons after he was seen on two separate occasions by doctors at the speedway - doctors who lacked the kind of familiarity with Hamlin that a personal care physician could provide."*

> *"If NASCAR is going to empower a medical professional to make decisions about whether a driver can race, it should be someone the driver already has a relationship with."*

> *"NASCAR says safety is a top priority. ... consistent medical staff would be good. ... The drivers need to know that, if they seek treatment, they'll receive care and guidance from a trusted doctor."*

> *"There's a big difference in seeing a doctor for the first time and visiting your regular physician - not only a sense of familiarity but a comfort in knowing the person understands your history."*

And of course, I wondered:

- *How did these racing teams comprehend the essential need for continuity, relationship, and trust to ensure safety?*
- *How did racing teams understand more than many healthcare leaders and policy makers?*

- *And how and what can we learn from these teams as we continue our efforts to improve the broken healthcare system?*

I also recognized that the members of these racing teams are patients and families too. Both in the literal sense that they are patients of the healthcare system and members of their families . . . but also that in the context of the racing team - the driver on these teams is essentially the patient and the other team members are his/her family.

And as such (using both lenses), these patients and families recognize that the current healthcare system (both within NASCAR and in the larger context) is not providing those essential factors that best position patients for optimal health and safety; i.e., continuity, relationship, and trust. And that doing so is essential to increase patient safety.

That said, there are some healthcare leaders and policy makers who do understand how critical these factors are and who are also working to evolve the healthcare system to ensure these factors are ever-present and having an impact. In fact, I was blessed to be part of the National Quality Forum's (NQF) Patient and Family Engagement Action Team where we recognized the following factors essential for optimal healthcare provision and patient safety:

1. *Relationship*
2. *Partnership*
3. *Respect*
4. *Trust*
5. *Listening*
6. *Stories*
7. *Inclusion*
8. *Collaboration*
9. *Empathy*
10. *Understanding*

. . . and in so doing, we developed an action pathway to ensure each patient and family is honored, preferences are understood, and that authentic partnerships between patients and families and care teams are developed to support each patients' life and health goals and to ensure patient safety.

Questions

1. As a healthcare leader or clinician, how are you ensuring continuity, relationship, and trust (partnership) is ever-present throughout the healthcare system?

    a. As healthcare leaders, doctors, nurses, and staff, how are you ensuring patients and families are honored and safe?

2. As a patient or family member, what is your role in this process, what are the barriers you are facing to creating partnerships with your clinician, and what would you recommend to improve the safety of patients?

Chapter 37

Clean Shaven

A week later, Doc and I were back in the hospital.

"I miss the kids."

"I know. They miss you, too. Tommy said he can't wait to play Batman with you. Haylee says she wants to play Pretty Pretty Princess, and Sammy said she can't wait to give you a hug."

"Mr. Dahlborg, my name is Cassie. And you are?"

"Darlene. Tom's wife."

"Nice to meet you. I am going to prepare Tom for this procedure. We need to shave the area of the incision site."

"Where will that be?" I asked.

"The incision will be made in your groin area," came Cassie's reply.

So, you need to shave my groin? I thought. *Ugh.*

"Mrs. Dahlborg, you can step out if you would like?"

"No. I will stay right here. Thank you."

Only slightly embarrassing to have your groin shaved by a women other than your wife, with your wife right in the room, I thought as I laid on the gurney exposed, vulnerable, being shaved in a very personal place by a person I have now known for less than two minutes.

Could this be done any differently, I thought, again trying to bring my focus away from myself. I am not sure. But having a clearer understanding of what needs to take place, how to best prep, and options all ahead of time would be a nice start.

"There you go. How was that?"

Actually, I had no idea how to answer that question.

"We will come in to get you shortly to wheel you to the operating room. Mrs. Dahlborg, when Tom is taken away, I will show you where you can wait if you like."

"That would be great."

And true to Cassie's word a few moments later and …

"Mr. Dahlborg, we are here to bring you to the surgical suite. Are you all set?"

Of course, I thought, *now that my groin is clean shaven I am.* But I knew that I was extremely tired and worn out and should just smile and keep my mouth shut.

"I will be waiting for you. I love you. You are going to be fine."

"I love you too, Darlene."

God that sounded weird, I thought. *I barely ever call Doc by her given name. But I just felt it made sense at this moment to do so rather than explaining to one of the doctors I have never met that I actually did not love them. That would just make things awkward.*

It is truly fascinating where your mind goes at times of stress. Or at least where my mind went.

It wasn't long before I was strapped down (or at least it felt that way) in the extremely cold surgical suite.

"Mr. Dahlborg, I am Dr. Granger. I am the anesthesiologist …"

I know he said a lot more, but for the life of me even at the time, I had no idea what he was saying. All I remember was …

"I can feel a stabbing in my groin."

"No, Mr. Dahlborg. You are not feeling anything."

"But I am. I can feel a stab …"

Later that afternoon …

"Tom. Tom. I am right here. They said you did great. It is all over. You are safe. You came back to me."

REFLECTION

"I went to see my physical therapist in an effort to avoid shoulder surgery. When I arrived, I learned my therapist would be treating me along with three other patients. She would instruct me to do an exercise, and when she could, would turn and rush over to another patient to correct that individual's form prior to doing the same with another, before making her way back to me to correct me as well. Of course, clearly I had been doing my rehabilitation incorrectly (as had my patient peers). I was not engaged but rather scared that I was doing more harm. My therapist was kind, but the system is broken and she was not helpful. I ended up having shoulder surgery, which at first felt beneficial, but now that pain is back, my work is in jeopardy and my doctor wants me to begin therapy again."

– Local small business owner and patient

"Payer X is reducing reimbursements for my patient visits significantly. I currently see each of my patients one-on-one for a full hour. My patients are engaged and activated. I focus on the whole person. We talk. We discuss what is working for them and what is not. We co-create their treatments. And my focus is 100 percent on their care and on supporting their recovery. This reduction in payment level is a barrier to optimal care provision and would lead to harm for my patients. Patient safety would be compromised due to lack of attention from having to see multiple patients at same time; patients will be placed in harm's way and could end up being over-treated (having unnecessary surgery due to lack of progress in rehab); and patients will be disengaged. I will not practice this way."

– Local physical therapist

Plan, Do, Study, Act–otherwise known as PDSA in quality-improvement speak–is critical to continuous improvement.

More specifically, PDSA refers to:

- ***Plan**: the change to be tested or implemented*

- ***Do**: carry out the test or change*

- ***Study**: data before and after the change and reflect on what was learned*

- *Act: plan the next change cycle or full implementation*

Albert Einstein reportedly said that the definition of insanity is doing the same thing over and over again and expecting different results.

If we tie this to quality improvement, insanity would be skipping the "study" aspect of improvement and thus not reflecting, learning, or improving.

Why do I share these stories and these two points here?

When faced with the need to reduce healthcare costs, healthcare finance leaders often mandate arbitrary unit cost reductions to decrease medical expense and improve the bottom line.

And yet arbitrary unit cost reductions, although they could positively impact financial results in the short term, do not lead to improved care outcomes, and in fact may actually increase long-term healthcare costs through patient harm and overtreatment.

The examples above are missing a crucial piece: Finance leaders and their healthcare delivery counterparts working collaboratively to develop creative approaches to care provision rather than simply dictating unit cost reductions.

In not doing so, they are (we all are) missing great opportunities to leverage quality improvement and person centeredness to develop models and programs that lead to appropriate care, improved outcomes and overall improved medical costs savings for the entire health system. (Savings that can be used to benefit others in need).

As healthcare finance leaders–be it within a hospital, managed care organization or other– we are part of a system and a community. We should have the same mission and vision within each of our healthcare institutions as the CEO, the doctors, the nurses, and the entire community in which we serve. And if short-term financial returns that place our patients, families and communities in harm's way is part of our mission, it is a shameful one and must be changed immediately. If it is not, we need to apply quality improvement and other innovative approaches to our work and join the efforts to create optimal care provision with new, innovative and financially responsible care models aligned with the quadruple aim. Only then will we truly both honor our mission and create a sound organization and system that truly serves all those in need.

Questions

1. As a clinician, have you ever felt pressured to provide care that is unnecessary? Please share your story.

2. As a clinician, have you ever felt pressured to withhold care that would benefit your patient? Please share your story.

3. As a patient, to your knowledge have you ever received unnecessary treatments? Please share your story.

4. As a patient, to your knowledge have you ever not received care you believed was essential to your health? Please share your story.

5. What would you recommend to fix this brokenness?

Chapter 38

Unnecessary

A week later, with still no improvement in my condition, Doc and I were back at my primary care physician's office.

"So Tom, you had a cardiac catheterization?"

"Yes, Dr. Schmidt said it would confirm my diagnosis."

"I have the results right here. The biopsy of your heart tissue is negative."

"That is a good thing, right?" I said as I looked from Dr. Iuvenis to Doc and then back to Dr. Iuvenis.

"Tom, it means the heart tissue that was analyzed looked normal."

At this, Dr. Iuvenis turned away from Doc and me and walked to the other side of the small exam room.

I looked to Doc pleading with my eyes as to what that meant.

Doc looked back to me and then over to Dr. Iuvenis who was now carrying a small office chair toward the two of us.

"A heart biopsy can correctly pinpoint a specific diagnosis in 10%-20% of cases," Dr. Iuvenis began as he sat on his chair which was now directly in front of us.

I made a mental note that this was one of the very few times any of my physicians sat so proximate to us and actually looked into our eyes for more than a fleeting moment.

"Are you saying," of course I knew the answer to the question I was about to ask but in my effort to grasp what I was hearing I asked it anyway, "that in 80%-90% of the cases, the cardiac cath that I had will not correctly pinpoint a specific diagnosis?"

I could almost read Doc's mind, "You [the healthcare system] worried me half to death, doing an invasive procedure on my husband that only works ten to twenty percent of the time? And with all the negative things that could have happened to my husband?!?!?!?"

By the way, Doc confirmed my assumption on our ride home.

Dr. Iuvenis turned in his chair and faced me directly as he responded to my question, "Yes, Tom. That is correct…"

It looked to me that he was about to say more so I waited. But no, he did not.

"What do we do now?"

"Darlene," Dr. Iuvenis was now turned toward Doc. "Tom has a follow up appointment scheduled with Dr. Schmidt, correct?"

"Yes, tomorrow," I interjected.

"Dr. Schmidt will also have these results and will share next steps with you."

"So, do I have viral myocarditis, Dr. Iuvenis?"

"Tom, everything points to that diagnosis."

"Except the cardiac cath results that are correct 10% to 20% of the time?" I said, unfortunately with a bit of sarcasm.

"That is correct, Tom."

"Then what do I do?"

"Meet with Dr. Schmidt and he will tell you what to do. He will give you a plan. Be patient Tom. It takes time."

Be patient? I am tired of being patient. I am tired of being a patient, I wanted to scream. *I also just had an invasive procedure that took its toll on my wife and kids and it is only accurate 10% to 20% of the time. And worst of all … no one told us those odds. Doc and I were uninformed and agreed to a procedure that if the data were known I believe we would not have proceeded.*

Up to this point I had worked in healthcare for almost fifteen years, and my bride was an amazing nurse, and neither of us during the stress of hearing an unpleasant (to say the least) diagnosis asked about the odds of success of a recommended invasive procedure. We should have known better. But what about those folks with no medical or healthcare understanding? What about those people with limited understanding of the English language never mind healthcare terminology? What about those who are elderly or poor or mentally or emotionally compromised? There has got to be a better way!

I looked at Doc and could see the Brockton rising in her chest.

And I could feel it in myself as well, *Damn it! I should have known better. I should not have put my bride through this. And I need to get well and help fix this.*

"I understand, Dr. Iuvenis. I do. But this is not easy. This has been going on for so long. My chest still hurts. I still feel like someone is constantly sitting on it. I am still tired all the time. My cough, my breathing, my head … I don't feel better at all."

"Stay on your current protocol from Dr. Schmidt. See him tomorrow. Get your updated plan from him. Be patient, Tom…"

Easy for you to say, was all I could think as my level of testiness continued to grow.

"… and keep me posted."

Doc and I were both clearly edgy on the ride back to Scarborough. She was chomping on the inside of her cheek as I stared out the van window as the pressure in my chest threatened to explode.

And between you and me, so did my temper. I was losing it. And of all people to lose it with, I did not want it to be the woman who has supported me with all of her heart and soul for so very long.

So, I turned my anger at God.

People throughout the world have it far worse than me. I get it. I get it. And even if I am to die, I have had an amazing thirty-five years on this earth. An incredible wife and three beautiful children inside and out. I get it. I have no right to be mad.

Yes, my mind was challenged. My fatigue at its peak. My heart broken physically and more. And I was yelling in my own mind at God.

The healthcare system is so broken. Doc and I are privileged in so many ways. We have so much in our favor to manage the system… and we are failing. Bureaucracies, paperwork, information being lost, access issues, confusion, fear, unnecessary treatment …

"Tom, did you want to stop at Dunks for an iced coffee?"

It took me a few moments to come back to the present and of course my response was a resounding, "YES!"

"Tom, do you want a large?"

Did she even need to ask?

REFLECTION

"Do you remember the show 'Name That Tune'?"

I did, of course, but also wondered why a cardiologist would be posing this question to me.

I had received the following message from the cardiologist in question:

> *"I've given my whole life to trying to put the patient first and would love to know if you are aware of any ways in which I could use my education and experience to further the cause."*

And over the next couple of months, she continued to share:

> *"You know I have always been passionate about patient care, but if possible, I am more so now."*

> *"I have seen 'healthcare' from so many different viewpoints and pray that my recent further eye-opening role as a patient will be of some benefit in reforming what appears to be a system in continual decline."*

> *"I found myself in my own ER recently and couldn't have conceived of a more pathetic interaction in a room where I'd stood so many times before. I know that you need to have 'connection' to the patient, but that can't be done in 5 minutes."*

During this time, we discussed the flames of goodness in healthcare and the challenges, many of them significant, before us.

We discussed Dr. Pam Wible's work relative to physician abuse and suicide.

We discussed the importance of relationship and trust in healing and at the end of life.

We discussed innovative new tools that could better position patients as they enter the complexity of the healthcare system.

And the sharing was inspiring as hearts and minds connected to better the system for others.

But back to "Name that Tune" ...

This wonderful physician went on to share that some years ago she left a group practice where the other physicians were literally betting each other that upon entering a new patient's exam room how quickly (in minutes) they could be in and out and on to the next patient.

"I can be in and out of the patient's room in 8 minutes."

"Well, I can be in and out in 7 minutes."

And so on and so on ... just like "Name That Tune."

Yes, regardless of the circumstances that brought the patient and family to the clinic that day, regardless of the information in the patient's electronic health record, the patient's prior test results or the socioeconomic factors that may be a key driver of his or her health concern, regardless of the patient's emotional condition, mental health challenges, health literacy, cultural background, the root cause of the health concern, the patient's support system, financial considerations, etc. ... regardless of the patient, these clinicians had their approach and would apply this same approach as quickly as possible.

And they would maximize revenues in doing so.

Efficient? Perhaps, using strictly a short-term impact lens.

Effective? Well, let's define our aim first. To maximize revenue? Apparently—or at least in the eyes of the physician practice owners.

But was the model effective in preventing overtreatment, keeping patients safe, improving patient experience, engaging patients, creating a safe space for relationship and trust to develop and to truly listen to and understand the patient's whole story, providing compassion and empathy, and producing optimal clinical outcomes?

At this point, let's simply say that these betting physicians lost many of their patients to my new cardiologist friend. Yes, they lost many patients to the physician who shared time with her patients, listened to their stories, and leveraged this new understanding of her patient with her own clinical wisdom and evidenced-based medicine to co-create a care path aligned with optimal care, patient safety, and the patient's preferences.

Questions

1. As a clinician, how important is it to share the odds of success of a treatment?

    a. How important is it for your patient to understand the odds?

2. As a healthcare leader, what processes have you put in place to ensure understanding?

3. As a patient or family member, what do you see your role is in ensuring an optimal understanding of your treatment plan?

4. What would you recommend to improve understanding throughout the system?

Chapter 39

Surrender

Over the next few months, Doc and I continued to face the challenges of maneuvering through the healthcare system. Be it continuing to obtain referrals from Dr. Iuvenis to see Dr. Schmidt, or manually carrying my medical record from Dr. Schmidt to Dr. Iuvenis to additional specialists and back again, to challenges faced with the phone systems throughout the healthcare system where the sparseness of human contact blatantly hits you in the face as you seek a reassuring voice when scared or in pain (be it Doc or myself) but only get a recording … each stop to seek care, to seek caring, continued to be painful. And it simply did not need to be.

And as time continued to pass and I continued to not see improvement in my health, my hopes and thoughts relative to returning to work and helping to fan the flame of what was good in the system and fix what was broken continued to decrease.

Until …

"Tom, there is no more we can do for you."

Doc and I had seen Dr. Schmidt almost weekly over the past few months. And today he was telling me like it was. Or at least like he saw it.

"Tom, we have done everything we can do. You have followed the plan I laid out perfectly, and that is it. Now you need time. Rest and time."

"But I need to get well for my family."

In my heart I was actually saying, "But I need to be a husband and a father again. For months I have let me family down. I have caused harm to my wife and children. I have become a burden."

I then turned to, "I need to get back to work. People are counting on me."

"Tom, I don't believe you will ever work again. And you should anticipate at some point the potential of requiring a heart transplant."

Although I had researched on many occasions the treatment for viral myocarditis and have read about the possibility for a heart transplant, hearing MY doctor confirm it all as he said this out loud in front of my wife decimated me.

"Doctor, that is rare, right?"

I spoke up having seen the look on Doc's face. Her eyes wider than I have ever seen, her mouth not chewing but rather open with no sound emanating.

"We need to be clear with one another, Tom. Your prognosis is not good. Your symptoms have not improved. You are still experiencing chest pressure and pain; you remain severely fatigued."

"But doctor, I will do anything."

Yes, I tried to negotiate with my cardiologist.

"Just tell me what to do. Please!"

"Tom, as I said, big picture at this point is the time and rest. But to help alleviate your pain I am sending you to the pain clinic at Brighton."

Pain clinic? Having had much experience with Percocet, Demerol, Tylenol with codeine, Darvocet, Vicodin, and I am sure other drugs from all of my orthopedic procedures, I was not interested in any more pain medications.

"But doctor, I would rather live with the pain and pressure than be medicated. I want to be me not a clouded me."

"Listen, Tom. You even said you want to get back to your family. A person in constant pain is not themselves. And I am sure you always hurting is stressing your wife and children. Let's get you some relief so you can be closer to the real Tom."

The real Tom? Who was he again?

This was not what I wanted to hear. In fact, none of this was. *Heart transplant? Not working again? Drugs? God, you and I have a lot to fight about later!* I screamed in my head as the tears began to stream down my face.

"Doc?"

"I want you out of constant pain." And then after a breath, "I think you should continue to follow Dr. Schmidt's plan."

Seeing the hurt and pain and surrender in Doc's face, I knew I couldn't say no.

REFLECTION

Every time I turn on the television, go to a bookstore or see a movie advertisement it seems I see "ZOMBIES." Zombies are everywhere. (Even the Centers for Disease Control and Prevention got into the action with its Zombie attack preparedness manual.)

Now I love zombie movies as much as anyone. In fact, "Shaun of the Dead" is one of my favorites, truly illustrating an existentialist view of life where people operate on autopilot.

After my most recent visit to the bookstore and the most recent zombie reminder, I got to thinking about people operating on autopilot. I have heard on many occasions from physicians and nurses alike that the traditional medical model–with the clinical guideline adherence; the relative value unit generation requirement; the constant goal of "fill in the box on the EMR," determine diagnosis, prescribe and get to the next patient as quickly as possible–contributes to the feeling of "practicing on autopilot" with little connection to self and/or patient (a zombie-like trance).

It's not that they don't want the connection. In fact, they share that they are desperate for the bond and long to reconnect with why they became healers in the first place.

Interestingly, being on autopilot is not restricted to only practitioners in healthcare. In a recent conversation with a public health official (an administrator) I heard the following: "I don't have time to think. I only have time to do. I have so much to do that even the thought of taking a moment to breathe and think about what I am doing, why I am doing it, and how to do it better ... just couldn't happen." Now this individual is a passionate, creative, caring person whose greatest gifts are being lost to the system as she transforms into a zombie-like state in an effort to "get things done."

In this same realm, a well-connected consultant was discussing quality of care with a CEO of a large hospital (who also happened to be a physician). The CEO discussed pressures — financial pressures — and responded to a question about improving care quality with the following: "Quality improvement focused on quality of care? I don't have time to focus on quality of care. I need to focus on improving efficiencies and revenue generation if I am to keep my hospital open. That is my focus. Care quality must take a backseat for now."

Care quality taking a backseat to fiscal pressures? It's another example of a caring, passionate, mission-driven healer/administrator being transformed by the broken healthcare system (with its misaligned financial drivers and intentions) into a zombie-like state with a limited focus on the bottom-line.

I was also fortunate to connect with a brilliant health IT consultant who shared the following story with me: "I had decided that the next primary care physician I selected must use an electronic medical record. I believed that optimal care would best be supported by a physician accessing an EMR. I made my new selection recently and went in for my initial visit. My new doctor had access to a plethora of my historical data. He could have seen trends in my blood pressure. He could have seen my prescription history, correlated what had a positive impact with what did not, and much more. But he did none of it. He did not have time. He asked me a couple of questions, he filled in the EMR boxes, and I was on my way. We had little discussion, little connection. The EMR had little positive impact. Now I have rethought my selection criteria and will find a physician who will connect with ME ... not only with the EMR ME."

Another physician on autopilot?

Can physicians in zombie-like states best position patients for optimal healing and patient safety? Can healthcare administrators showing zombie-like tendencies best position clinicians to provide optimal care and safety?

Absolutely not!

My evidence? Look at the patients who are being harmed by the system. Look at the adverse events and errors in care provision. Look at the patients the system is giving up on. Autopilot does not work.

As I began to write this reflection, I happened upon an older blog titled: "Heroes Not Zombies." To my pleasant surprise rather than reading about "brain eaters" I saw the blog post "The importance of the doctor patient relationship." And according to the post, "Relationships are fundamental to happiness. And so a science that has the courage to include the doctor's relationship with the patient within the treatment itself, and to work with it, is a science already modeling the solution it prescribes."

The healthcare system must change.

The healing encounter must evolve to include optimal time for connection, relationship, trust, empathy and must do so in conjunction with quality improvement, optimal technology and care systems all being best leveraged to improve care (not predominantly for revenue generation).

Practitioners must be allowed to turn off the autopilot switch, reconnect with themselves, their passion for healing, their patients, and the reason they became healers in the first place.

And us administrators, we also must reconnect with ourselves, our passions, the reason we got into healthcare ... and if we determine we are here for any reason other than improving the health and lives of our friends, our neighbors, our families and our communities, then we ought to move on.

It is time to stem the tide of the healthcare zombie epidemic. Are you ready?

Questions

1. As a healthcare leader or clinician, when was the last time you were NOT on autopilot? How did it feel? Please share that story.

2. As a clinician or patient, have you ever felt a sense of hopelessness? What did you do? Please share your story.

Chapter 40

The Menu

After continued challenges with referrals, phone systems, ensuring my primary care physician was in the loop and my insurer willing to pay, I finally made my way to the pain clinic at Brighton.

"Mr. Daltrub …"

"Dahlborg. Tom Dahlborg."

"Oh yes. Mr. Dahlborg. I am Dr. Albert. How are you today?"

'How are you?' has become one of those questions I never want to hear again.

"I am okay."

"Well, certainly you are not if you are here at the pain clinic."

See?

"Well, Tom, here is the deal. This is your menu."

Dr. Albert was now holding a three-ring binder in front of me.

"This is your list."

It was a list of narcotics.

"Just tell me where you would like to start."

"Excuse me?"

"I am here to help relieve you of your discomfort. These medications are tools in this process. This is a list of all of your tools."

"Okay."

My fatigue was clearly setting in. And through a cloud of exhaustion I pointed to the first opiate on the list.

That evening I opted to not take the first dose of my new medication.

"Tom, you will feel better. You will finally get relief. You will finally get some good sleep. Honey, you need to take your meds."

"Doc, I am just not ready. I can't."

God, how I hate letting Doc down. God, how I hate saying 'I can't'! I silently yelled upward.

The next morning was no different. And yet, for Doc, I knew I needed to try. I knew I needed to take my medicine. And, yes, the phrase 'take my medicine' was not lost on me.

And so, I did. Without telling Doc, without making a big deal outwardly, although inwardly it was a huge deal to me, early the next morning I took the first dose.

"'morning Daddy."

"Good morning, Tommy."

Although thirty minutes after my first dose, the morning was not feeling good at all.

"Can I have some cereal?"

Jesus, Tommy. I am tired. Can't you wait? I thought as my son with his innocent blue eyes and beautiful smile looked up at me.

"Daddy! Can I have some cereal?" Tommy repeated.

"Yes!" I responded as I stomped my way to the kitchen.

"Daddy, I want Rice Krispies this morning," Tommy said melodically as I was bent over in the closet.

"Daddy, I want Rice Krispies!" Tommy said again with his sweet lyrical voice as I continued to hunt down the elusive Rice Krispies box hiding apparently in plain sight.

"Daddy …"

"TOMMY!! …

YOU NEED TO BE PATIENT!!! …

HERE IS YOUR FUCKING CEREAL!! ...

TAKE IT! TAKE IT!! TAKE IT!!!" I yelled as a beast from within my heart and soul burst through and took over.

"GET THE FUCK AWAY FROM ME! GET THE FUCK AWAY FROM ME!! GET THE FUCK AWAY FROM ME!!!" I screamed as, for the first time in a very long time, I ran ... after throwing the cereal box at the wall, I ran from the kitchen down the short hallway and into the bathroom.

"Tom! Tom! Tom!" I could hear coming from the stairway as I slammed the bathroom door shut and fell into the wall on my way to the floor.

"My God! My God! My God! What did I just do? My God!!"

"Tom! Tom! What happened? What happened? Tom! Open this door! Open this door!"

Oh my God! Oh my God! I can't do this. I can't do this. I hurt my son, I chanted over and over.

"Tom. Tom. Listen to me. Listen to me. You are okay. You are okay. Listen to me. You are okay. Open this door."

Please God. Please, I prayed as I reminded myself to breathe.

"Please Tom. Open this door. Tommy is fine. Open this door."

"Doc," I whispered through the shut door. "I can't do this anymore. I can't."

"What Tom? What can't you do?"

"Any of it. I can't ..."

I paused as I wiped the mixture of sweat and tears off of my face and caught my breath.

Doc was silent.

"Doc, I can't fight anymore," I whispered. And then, "And I can't take these drugs. I can't Doc. I can't be this way."

"Tom. Listen to me," Doc began so very calmly. "You don't have to take the drugs anymore. We will flush them right now if you want. You don't have to. Open this door, and we will flush them together. Do you hear me? We will flush them together."

REFLECTION

After recently hearing about the latest spate of deaths due to the opioid epidemic along with the news that one of Rocky Marciano's relatives from Brockton (and an amazing athlete in his own right, who also happened to be tough as nails) was also felled by this disease, I look back at the path that was before me and think, "But for the Grace of God go I."

Opioid Prescribing Practices

- In 2014, more than 240 million prescriptions were written for prescription opioids, which is more than enough to give every American adult their own bottle of pills. Raising further alarm, four in five new heroin users started out by misusing prescription opioids.
- The Centers for Disease Control and Prevention (CDC) in March 2016 released its Guideline for Prescribing Opioids for Chronic Pain to provide recommendations for the prescribing of opioid pain medication for patients 18 and older in primary care settings.
- As of March 2016, CDC has awarded over $30 million to 29 states to improve safe prescribing practices, such as enhancing Prescription Drug Monitoring Programs (PDMPs), through its Prescription Drug Overdose (PDO) grants. CDC has recently released a funding announcement, which could expand to 50 states by the end of FY 2016.
- In January 2016, the Centers for Medicare and Medicaid Services (CMS) released an Informational Bulletin on Medicaid best practices for addressing prescription drug overdoses, misuse and addiction.
- In October 2015, the Administration announced that over 40 provider groups committed to training prescribers in safe prescribing. Since then, more than 60 medical schools and 191 nursing schools have committed to requiring their students to take some form of prescriber education in line with the CDC Guideline.
  Source: The Opioid Epidemic: By the numbers; Department of Health and Human Services, June 2016

On an average day in the U.S.:
- More than 650,000 opioid prescriptions dispensed
- 3,900 people initiate nonmedical use of prescription opioids
- 580 people initiate heroin use
- 78 people die from an opioid-related overdose

Economic Impact of the Opioid Epidemic:
- 55 billion in health and social costs related to prescription opioid abuse each year
- 20 billion in emergency department and inpatient care for opioid poisonings

Source: Pain Med. 2011;12(4):657-67.1 2013;14(10):1534-47.2 1. CDC, MMWR, 2015; 64;1-5. 2. CDC Vital Signs, 60(43);1487-1492 *Opioid-related overdoses include those involving prescription opioids and illicit opioids such as heroin Source: IMS Health National Prescription Audit1 / SAMHSA National Survey on Drug Use and Health2 / CDC National Vital Statistics System3

Questions

1. As a healthcare leader or clinician, what do you see as the key drivers of the opioid epidemic?

    a. What role has financially incentivizing patient experience and patient satisfaction scoring played in the epidemic?

2. As a clinician, what improved training have you received in opioid prescribing? How would you improve this training?

3. As a clinician, how do we ensure we best position patients and families to manage pain without exacerbating the opioid epidemic?

    a. What other non-medicinal approaches to pain management would you recommend?

4. As a healthcare leader or clinician, what system improvements are required to address?

    a. What changes have you made in your organization to address this challenge?

    b. If you have not made any changes, what barriers stand in the way? What would you recommend to break down these barriers?

5. As a patient and/or family member, how has this impacted your life? Please share your story.

Chapter 41

Resignation

"Doc, I need to. It is the right thing to do."

"Oh, honey. I know. I know. We will be fine. We will be fine."

"Good morning, Saul."

"Tom! It is so great to see you. How are you feeling? We miss you around here!"

"That is why I am here, Saul."

"First come into my office and have a seat. You look exhausted."

I followed Saul into his office overlooking Casco Bay. The sun was reflecting off the water cascading prisms of light off the cars in the parking lot and into my eyes. Squinting, I thought about this place. This flawed and amazing organization with a mission to take care of people. With a mission to take care of those who have protected and served this nation.

A tear began to roll down my face as I thought about loss.

Loss and losing.

The loss of an opportunity to help make things better. To serve my team and my patients and members. Like a break up with someone you truly love, when you realize that it actually was not meant to be, I felt that hollowness in my gut as if cupid somehow morphed into a plow horse and kicked me just above my belt line. Even more alone I felt as if a great love was being taken from me and no matter how much I yearned, how much I tried, how much I begged and pleaded and planned and worked, it was not meant to be.

My great love was being taken away, and I was helpless.

My great love was being taken away, and I was in pain.

My great love was being taken away, and I hurt.

My great love was being taken away, and now I must surrender and walk away myself.

I was provided with a great opportunity to make a difference, and I could not.

Someone once said that it is better to have loved and lost than to never have loved before. They were wrong. My love had pulled my wife and children away from our family in Massachusetts. My love had set expectations I now could not deliver on. My love had set an expectation for Mrs. Jones and her husband, and all my patients and members I sought to help, that a difference would be made … and now I was abandoning them worse off because now they, too, will feel a loss. They, too, will know what it feels like to be let down and left behind.

God, this hurts so badly. I don't want to lose my love. I don't want to fail. I don't want to do more harm to the already broken system.

"How can I be in so much torment in such a wondrous location?" I asked the Universe as I took a seat across from Saul.

"Saul, I have been soul searching."

"Tom, can I get you a tissue?"

Clearly my attempt to hide my heart was to no avail. Yes, my head although pounding was engaged, but so was my heart. My broken heart. Yes, broken in so many ways.

"Thank you, Saul," I tried to joke. "Clearly I need it."

"Saul …" I swallowed hard as I tried to hold back all of the pain.

"Tom, you said you have been soul searching. What is troubling you?"

Okay, Tom, I thought as I continued to breathe, hold back tears, and process how best to say what I was about to say, *You can do this. Clearly, slowly, calmly, just say it. Just do it.* And yes, my own internal reference to a NIKE commercial almost made me smile.

"Yes, Saul. You and my entire team have been so ethereal to me."

Of course, I wondered where that word came from.

"From your help with my seeking care, to Sandy and others sending over meals, to the cards, and flowers …"

I almost could not even say the words as my heart once again felt the love that so many had shared with me and my family. The care that I wanted for all of our patients and members was shown to me by my awe-inspiring team and others.

And then again my mind went to the dark place of, "and now I am abandoning them after they have done so much for me."

"We do have a wonderful team, don't we?"

"We sure do, Saul. We sure do."

Phew, a respite, I thought. And then, *Okay, back to business. Time to 'rub some dirt on it' as my Dad would say.*

"Saul, I have soul searched. And yes, the team has been incredible in so many ways. And you have been so supportive. First, I want to thank you. You have no idea what you and all you have done has meant to me and my family. From the bottom of my [broken] heart," and then almost in an inaudible whisper I somehow managed to get out, "thank you."

"Tom," Saul began as I grabbed another tissue, "you mean a lot to us."

"Saul," I continued, "I love this place. I love our mission."

"I know you do, Tom. We all know you do."

Wow, that meant a lot coming from Saul.

"Saul, it is unfair to you, unfair to my team, and unfair to all those we serve for there not to be a leader in the COO role in place and present."

"Tom, you are the COO."

Okay, that one I must admit caught me off guard, but I knew that even though I was dying here I needed to continue.

"Yes, but for a long time I have not been honoring my commitments. And Saul, my prognosis is not good."

"What are you saying, Tom?"

As I grabbed for more tissues and the tears begin to stream down my face, "Saul, I am resigning as the COO. I am not doing the job. I cannot do the job. As I said, it is unfair to everyone for so much to be on hold as people wait for me. It is wrong, and I cannot ask people to do that anymore. I am so sorry for all of this. But I know that me stepping aside is the right thing to do."

Saul was truly great as I found I could not say much more at this point. I had just told a great love I needed to move on (whatever that was going to look like) and now physically and mentally exhausted and in pain, with my heart broken, I was wiped out and ready to go home and back on the couch which has served as my dock for so very long.

"Tom, Listen to me. You do not need to make this decision today. Clearly, you are going through a lot…"

"Saul, before you go on," I began to say with a strength I didn't think I still had in me, "I appreciate what you are about to say. But I know this is the right decision. I know that even though this hurts more than I ever thought it would, it is what is best. All I ask is permission to go and visit with my team this afternoon to tell them personally."

Again, Saul was so good to me. He listened, he was empathetic, he appropriately offered other options and, in the end, he truly heard and honored my preference.

"Thank you, Saul," I said completely exhausted.

"How are you going to get over to South Portland?"

Still caring, I thought.

"My bride is driving. She is in control. No worries."

"Tom, you look exhausted. I am taking you home. You can see your team another time."

Always taking care of me she was.

"No. Word travels too fast. I must see them now. They must hear from me directly that I am leaving."

"You listen to me. You mean more to me than that. You are coming home with me, and I am taking care of you. You are all that matters to me. You, Tom. I love YOU."

The love a man can feel for his soul mate is almost indescribable. Here I was, I have pulled my bride away from her family, especially her mother, and brought her up to Maine, to a land she thought was Alask-ian. To a location away from all her friends and support system. All for a position which I loved and touched my heart, mind and soul, but in which in the end I could not do.

And now we were planning to significantly downsize, to leave our beautiful home near the coast, and move to a smaller home in which we could afford on my bride's nursing salary.

And here was my bride still loving me with all she has, supporting me in ways we never thought would be necessary, and never giving an inch to what we now call "the monster," aka my illness.

Was there an upside in all this?

Yes, we have also seen amazing signs of empathy from our children. From Sammy holding me on the couch and sharing gestures of love, and best of all her hugs. To Tommy leaning his head onto my chest and letting me wrap my arms around his sturdy frame as he looked up into my worn face and asked if I am okay and can he help. To my Haylee curling up in my arms and simply resting with me as we talked about all the big events in her life.

And also, Angus, who had continued to remain by my side throughout this journey. There had been many a night when I had woken up on my couch from a nightmare and have shared all my fears and angst with God's little creature, things I have not shared with anyone else, and no matter what, Angus had never judged me or lost his ability to love me unconditionally.

Yes, mixed in with the chaos, fear, sadness, heartache, and loss, had been some of the most loving and now cherished experiences of my life. And each day, even though incredibly hard, I tried to hold onto these moments and feel them to my very soul. To remember the warm embrace married to the bear-like protection of my bride each time the healthcare system had let us down, to see the intense loving blue eyes of each of my children as they looked deeply into my tired eyes and professed their love for me in so many ways, to hold onto the feeling of the beating heart and warm fur of Angus as he cuddled with me and laid his head on my chest. Yes, I tried to remember all of these moments.

REFLECTION

"Tom, if I quit, I am quitting on my son. I am quitting on my community."

Alejandro's son was admitted to the intensive care unit of a local hospital. For bureaucratic (aka bizarre) reasons, Alejandro was not allowed to be with his son in the hospital. He did not know if his son would live or die. He was not allowed to hold his son. Touch his son. Talk to his son. His son was alone. And so was Alejandro.

"Over time my son was healed ... as was I."

Not being with his son when his son needed him most hurt Alejandro deeply and that hurt became anger.

"I was healed with great support from many. My anger, my hurt ... my heart was healed. And now I am whole again and will ensure that no other family will go through what I did."

Alejandro explained further why he volunteers as a Patient Family Advisor (PFA) at the hospital where his greatest hurt was realized.

"We need to help people. We need to have a good heart. We need to educate people. We are here for them. I am here for them. I don't want anyone to feel alone or to be alone. My work ethic and my love keeps me on this journey."

Be it a hospital, a school, a workplace, a home ... many people feel alone. Many people are alone. Some choose to be on occasion. Others are pushed into aloneness by bizarre rules with unintended (or intended) consequences.

Alejandro wrapped up our discussion with the following simple and powerful message, "I am going to stay and help others."

There are a great many lessons to be learned from adversity. We can become negative and fall in the blame game or we can learn and grow and make things better.

Alejandro makes things better for others every day.

Questions

1. As a healthcare staff person, patient or family member, what challenges have you faced that could have left you bitter?

    a. How did you overcome?

    b. How have you turned that experience into a blessing and an opportunity to benefit others?

    c. Please share your story.

Chapter 42

Goodbye

"No, Doc," I said with as much vigor as I could muster. "I need to talk to my team now. Please take me to my office."

"Tom," Doc began to say but I cut her off by putting my hand on her arm and looking deeply into her eyes while saying, "I need to do this, Doc. The harm to my body has already been done. This is the least I can do for my team. To tell them face-to-face."

I am uncertain if Doc did not respond because she was mad or because she was afraid of crying.

So I too, decided to simply remain quiet, catch my breath, and close my eyes as we made the ten-minute journey to the next chapter in our lives.

"Oh my gosh, Tom, you are back. It is so great to see you!"

"Thank you, Esther. It is great to see you, too."

"We have missed you so very much around here. People constantly are asking, 'How is Tom? When is he coming back?' and those types of things. Are you back? We have so much work to do!"

"Thanks, Esther," I wanted to say. Both from a genuine place of gratitude because the warm feelings being shared meant so very much to me and because I too wanted to be back … but it was not meant to be.

"Esther, I am here today to let you and the rest of our team know that I just resigned."

"Tom!" Esther began to say louder than I think she meant to as she placed her left hand over her mouth. But before she could say more, I continued…

"Esther, I have been told that at this time the healthcare system cannot do anything more for me."

"Oh Tom," but again she caught herself prior to continuing.

"I wanted to tell you all in person. I have already met with Saul and told him. At that time, I also shared some thoughts relative to next steps and some possibilities to ensure everything continues to move forward."

"I am so sorry, Tom. I didn't know."

"Please don't be." Now the words, like magic, were coming without any forethought on my part. "This is my journey to take. Mine and my families. We will be fine. It is me who is sorry. I am so sorry I could not support our team more. And I am truly sorry I will miss seeing the incredible impact you and our team (your team) will make."

Somehow, I was not crying. In fact, I felt as if I was out of my body watching as someone else remained so calm.

And for the next ninety minutes I circled the building, yes very slowly, and met with all of my direct reports and many of the other very special people all working together to make a difference.

"I am so going to miss these people," I thought to myself as I headed down the final hallway after spending the most time with my remarkable network development team.

Tom, I reminded myself as I continued my stroll, *never forget the feelings of love from all of these people.*

Clearly, they had concerns about new leadership and direction and the impact on each of them of this news and I am sure so much more, but not once was any of that mentioned. And, in fact, even when I offered to share more details in these spaces, no one took me up on it.

They all wanted to share their gratitude with me, I continued to process. *For me?* I was still amazed. *I have let them down. I am not able to lead them the rest of the way. And they are thanking me?*

Never forget.

"Oh Tom," Tory said when she saw me slowly approaching her cubicle. "I heard the news."

"Yes, Tory. I am so sorry."

"Now you listen here, young man..."

Although I believe we are close to the same age, for some reason Tory liked to refer to me as 'the kid.' And honestly, for some reason I liked it.

"I know you have been through a lot in the healthcare system. I know we …" Tory's reference to 'we' is as I have said before, 'we' have all had a role in creating the broken healthcare system, "… have failed you. But you are not giving up hope. Do you hear me?"

"God I love Brockton-tough nurses like my bride and sister," I remember thinking to myself as Tory continued to lecture me … out of love and concern.

It was hard for me to figure out how to respond so I simply looked up from my gaze at the floor and into her caring eyes.

"I know you have been through what appears to be the entire healthcare system. I know you have been put in danger with invasive procedures. I know you have had to carry your own medical record from doctor to doctor to doctor. I have this right, don't I?"

I have provided some updates to folks during this journey. And today, Tory was spot on.

"Yes, Tory."

"I am also betting many non-medical folks have provided you with exhaustive opinions on what you should do and not do. Right?"

"Yes, very well-meaning people have shared thoughts with me, Tory."

"I didn't say they were not well-meaning, did I?"

Oh yes, I love Brockton-tough nurses, I thought again as a small smile began to appear on my face.

"Oh, Tom. You have done so much good here."

Oh, how I needed to hear that this day.

"We all care so much about you."

It is amazing how healing gratitude is.

"And I know you. You are not giving up. You are simply taking a detour. I am right, aren't I?"

Really liking where she was going with this, I nodded my head. But honestly, I had been so tired, so scared, so down, the strength I felt months ago when I said to Doc, "I got this. Don't worry." That had been lost as more and more I realized that it didn't matter what I knew or who I knew, the healthcare system was profoundly broken, I contributed to its brokenness, and according to my doctors I was not going to get better.

But sitting here with Tory and truly accepting hers and my team's heartfelt responses to my news I began to feel a slight shift.

"Tory," I began to respond but she cut me off.

"Listen to me. I know you are in pain, and this is hard. But it is just a detour. Know that. It is just a detour. You are meant for more. You have supported and helped us in so many ways. Now it is your time to rest, heal, and follow a new path. You will be back. I know this. You will."

REFLECTION

To each who've wandered lost and small

He clears a path for you

Over and under and through the fear, he perseveres

Masculine and soft, vulnerable and brave, lion and mouse: he roars, protects-he sacrifices, surrenders

A beacon for so many, a leader, a coach, a lover, an artist, a believer, a father, a warrior of hope

So many things you are, so many things you will be.

(written by a good friend and servant leader)

Questions

1. As a healthcare leader, clinician, or staff person, do you know who those people are that will support you no matter what?

    a. And do those you would support in the same fashion know you are there for them?

    b. What can you do by next Tuesday to ensure your support system understands how truly important they are to you?

Chapter 43

A New Path

A few weeks later I was visiting with Tory again, and Tory the Coach was back at it.

"Now, Tommy, as I said last time, I know you have been through a lot and are tired and weary. But I need you. I need you to trust me. And I need you to step up. Will you do that?"

"What do you mean?"

My response was apprehensive for sure and yet, with the relationship Tory and I had developed, I trusted her.

"Dr. Ben Amare is an amazing physician in Falmouth. You will love him. You two are very much alike and he has developed a practice that aligns greatly with where you have been driving us. In fact, every time Tracie came back from the quality improvement work she has been doing with you and the rest of your team, she had shared many of the outputs with me and the rest of her staff. Not only was I completely bought in with the direction, I also noted that what you all are going to create is what Dr. Amare believes in and practices every day. So, long story short, you need to see him. He will help you on your new path."

As Tory was stressing these last points, she had left the chair behind her desk and was now kneeling in front of me with her hands in mine while looking into my eyes.

"Your new path, Tom." She repeated. "Your new path is a path you began to manifest here. Now it is time to follow it wherever it takes you. Understand?"

Later that afternoon Doc and I discussed my latest conversation with Tory and, like me, Doc was apprehensive.

"Ben Amare? Have you ever heard of him?"

"No, but rather than continuing to accept 'we cannot do anymore for you', Dr. Amare appears to be a new option with, according to Tory, a different approach. A new path." And then after an unintentional dramatic pause ala Tracie, "I figure I have nothing to lose at this point."

"Are you sure you want to see another doctor right now? I thought you wanted to take a break from the system for a while?"

"That is just it, Doc. Tory believes Dr. Amare will be a 'break from the broken healthcare system.'" And honestly, now that 'Coach' Tory shared what she did and the way she did, I have some hope plus..."

At this point I noticed I began to chew the side of my mouth. Perhaps I was trying to convince myself more than convince Doc.

"… a great deal of intellectual curiosity about Dr. Amare's approach. In fact, I am almost excited about it."

"Tom, I will do anything you want," Doc replied with a great deal of weariness both in her voice and body language.

"Doc, I want to follow a new path and get well again. I don't want to feel that I have let everyone down anymore, especially you and the kids. I want to come back from this and do good. Perhaps Dr. Amare is part of this. Perhaps, he is not."

"Hi, Yes. My name is Tom Dahlborg and I would like to schedule an appointment with Dr. Amare."

Even my initial contact with Dr. Amare's office was different. My call was answered by a human being within just a couple of rings. (There was no queue for incoming calls.) I was informed that I should plan for my initial visit with Dr. Amare to be about ninety minutes. And that I should ideally bring a trusted family member or friend with me.

Already I was curious as to his model and what I could learn.

"Doc, we have an appointment with Dr. Amare tomorrow at 9:30am. He wants to meet with you, too."

"They told you that over the phone?"

"Yes. And our appointment is scheduled from 9:30am until 11:00am."

"A ninety-minute appointment? Are you sure?"

"Oh yes. I confirmed it. This is going to be interesting at the very least."

"Tom, you look tired and are holding your chest again. Please go lay down."

I don't recall much of the rest of the day as I predominantly slept while still tethered to my couch.

But I do recall at least one of my three children and my pup with me at all times ensuring that I was okay.

"Daddy, do you like my dinosaur?"

"I sure do, T."

"Mommy says you are too tired to play with me. But Daddy," Tommy said as he looked first at my chest and then deeply into my eyes, "That is okay. You need to rest. I will just play here on the couch, and you can watch. How does that sound?"

"How about I play but just very slowly? Would that be okay, T?"

"Oh yes, Daddy," Tommy yelled as he jumped onto my lap and gave me a big bear hug. "You can have my yellow dinosaur with the little arms, and I will have my three horned dinosaur. Okay?"

"Perfect, T. Perfect."

And then as we played with our dinosaurs, I made mental note of the features of my son's face, his big innocent blue eyes, the 'm' of his ruby red upper lip, along with his wispy blond hair, huge shoulders and arms, and his 'little boy' voice as he said, "Daddy, I love you".

REFLECTION

"I'm a family doc in Eugene, Ore., where we've lost three physicians in 18 months to suicide. I was suicidal once. Assembly-line medicine was killing me. Too many patients and not enough time sets us up for failure."

There are many studies highlighting the harm our broken healthcare system does to patients–e.g., hospital errors occurring in one-third of all hospital admissions; medical mistakes contributing to up to 187,135 deaths and 6.1 million injuries; an estimated annual cost of measurable preventable medical errors of $17.1 billion (based on 2008 dollars).

But what about the harm caregivers face?

Many studies have highlighted the fact that physicians have a significantly elevated suicide rate in comparison to other professionals. In her article "What I've learned from saving physicians from suicide," Pamela Wible, M.D., highlights that not only are doctors overworked, exhausted and depressed, but few are seeking help.

A physician friend of mine from a well-known, local health care system confided in me that he was so tired and burned out that he was thinking of leaving the practice of medicine. As a primary care physician, he was feeling his role had moved further away from that of a healer and more toward a "production worker."

Rather than focus his energy on best positioning his patients for optimal healing, he was pressured to triple book every 15 minutes to generate the required 30 relative value units (RVU) per day and thus "earn" his salary.

He said he had lost his soul for healing. Today he spends most of his time on non-patient-care activities, doing medical claims reviews for a large insurer instead.

This represents another lost opportunity. Another lost primary care physician who would rather care for patients but not at the cost of his soul or his patient's safety.

Another friend of mine, at the time a resident physician, shared similar sentiments. Her residency program emphasized the need for speed (productivity) when it came to completing patient assessments, rather than ensuring patient safety and optimal outcomes.

She was tired, considered leaving the practice of medicine, and knew the broken healthcare system was not healthy for her or for her patients.

Back in 2008-2009, the Daniel Hanley Center for Health Leadership brought together healthcare leaders to improve primary care physician recruitment and retention in rural areas, and yet what we learned transcends beyond recruitment and retention to the soul of true healing.

We learned physicians are concerned with finding organizations that truly care about them. We learned physicians define the "caring" that they seek from organizations to entail:

> *» Finding an organization that is willing to create an optimal practice model that positions the physician to focus on healing (and not revenue generation) ... improving patient experience, safety and outcomes along with recruitment and retention of physicians.*
> *» Finding a practice that will develop support systems sensitive to the understanding of the physician's goals and needs ... helping to heal the healer prior to them leaving the primary care workforce (or worse).*
> *» Finding an organization with a commitment to collaboration and the creation and nurturing of a community of healers with a focus on learning, growing, sharing, supporting, and healing.*

Over the years and in my own experiences leading a medical practice, I have borne witness to this. I have heard physicians and others share how being loved, honored, and sometimes challenged in a trusted community has deepened their ability as healthcare providers, increased their confidence, courage and trust, and connected them more strongly with a sense of meaning in their work.

To truly honor the calling to serve our patients, we also must honor the calling of healing the healer. Only when caregivers are healthy (physically, mentally, emotionally, spiritually), and not pressured with harmful productivity requirements, will they (will we) be best positioned to improve patient experience, outcomes, safety and all truly heal.

Questions

1. As a healthcare leader, how much time do you allot for clinicians to spend with each of your patients?
2. As a clinician, how much time are you allotted to spend with each of your patients?
    a. How much time should you be sharing with your patients?
3. As a patient, do you feel you have enough time and undivided attention with your clinician?
4. What would you recommend to ensure optimal time is shared between patients and clinicians?
5. As a healthcare leader, what systems have you developed to ensure active and appropriate family engagement in healing?
6. As a clinician, how important to you is it that a family member or trusted friend participates in your patient's care journey?
7. As a patient, how important to you is it that a family member or trusted friend participates in your care journey?
8. What would you recommend to ensure appropriate family members and / or trusted friends are engaged?

Chapter 44

Together

"Why do you think Dr. Amare wants you to join me at my appointment?"

"Probably to find out the truth about you!"

She is good. And quick.

"All the times you don't listen to me. All the times you get broken because you don't listen to your body. He probably knows that you won't share all."

Doc then turned and looked at me as I laid my head onto the back of the couch.

"If you are going to get better," she caught herself, "when you get better, it will be because you start listening to me and to your body. Tom, I love you, but you overdo … everything. I believe this is a warning to you. A warning that you must start taking better care of yourself."

Doc's voice began to trail off and get softer, "I want you with us forever."

But she then finished with the fire I know and love, "So you WILL do what the Doctor says. And you WILL heal. Understand?"

I wasn't sure if she meant her as in 'Doc'- tor or Dr. Amare. Perhaps both and?

The ride to Falmouth seemed quite long. And even though Maine's traffic is nothing compared to a commute from the South Shore into Boston, it does still have its challenges. There was congestion getting out of Scarborough; Route One was always busy in the morning. And then 295 was slowed by an accident on the north side as folks 'rushed' to get to work or up to Freeport for shopping at L.L. Beans or one of the many outlets in the area.

"Don't worry, we will get there on time."

Doc knew me so well. I felt like I was heading to the first day of work at a new job and didn't want to be late.

"It's already twenty past nine, and we are still on 295."

"Don't worry. We will get there when we are supposed to."

No big deal for her, I thought. *This is not her first day on the job.*

I actually did see this as a job. The job to get well and whole again.

"Here is Exit 10. Not too far from here. Don't worry."

"Good morning."

"Good morning," I replied a bit winded after climbing with Doc's assistance up a number of dark carpeted stairs. "I am Tom Dahlborg, and I have an appointment with Dr. Amare at 9:30am today I believe."

"Oh yes, Tom. We spoke yesterday. I am Mary, Dr. Amare's assistant. I maintain his patient schedule, manage the billing, and help new patients get settled. I have some paperwork for you and Darlene to complete. Do I have that name right, Darlene?"

"Yes. I am Darlene, Tom's wife," Doc replied and then added, "Does Dr. Amare really want to see me, too?"

"Oh yes. If that is alright with the both of you of course."

"Hi, I am Dr. Amare. Ben Amare. You must be Darlene. And you must be Tom."

Dr. Amare came out of what appeared to be his office within a few minutes. In fact, perfect timing as Doc and I had just completed the office paperwork. He was about 5 feet 9 inches tall with dark brown hair, an easy smile, and a rock-hard handshake.

"Yes, I am Darlene." "And I am Tom." We both responded as we each stood up and shook Dr. Amare's outstretched hand.

"Wonderful. It is so very nice to meet you both. We will be meeting in my office in a moment. I just need to speak with Mary, and then I will be right with you."

And literally Dr. Amare was back with us within seconds and escorting us both into his office and to the two chairs lined up perpendicular to his desk.

As I sat, I noticed the room was fairly sparse. The walls were lightly painted, he had a couple of medical school diplomas and whatnot hanging on the wall behind him, an exam table on the other side of the room, and a large dark brown antique desk at which he was now sitting with his chair turned toward both Doc and me.

There was nothing between the three of us. No desk. No computer. Just the three of us sharing one space.

"A beautiful desk."

"Thank you. I purchased this antique just after medical school. It was both inexpensive and beautiful, so I figured I could not pass it up."

Doc and I both laughed.

"Doctor, I am not sure why I am here."

"Darlene. Is it okay if I call you Darlene?"

"Oh yes. Although if you hear Tom refer to 'Doc,' that is me too. A long story," Doc said through a big smile and her wonderful and distinctive laugh.

And laughing as well, Dr. Amare responded, "Well clearly Tom knew he needed a fulltime doctor."

"Oh, you don't know the half of it!"

"Doc, I am sitting right here," I interjected as we all laughed together.

"Well, I am sure we will get to that. But back to your question, Darlene. You would like to know why I asked you intentionally to join us for this visit."

Dr. Amare, wearing dark colored khakis and a light blue shirt with the sleeves rolled up and no tie, leaned over and placed his hands on his elbows, lowered his voice, and looked right into Doc's eyes, and continued, "From what I gather to date, we have a long road to hoe together. And I mean that … together. There will be challenges we expect and some we don't. And as we get to know one another and understand one another better, we will have a better sense for our different roles and responsibilities, along with the supports Tom will need and the supports you and your children will need. It is important that we develop a relationship where over time we will feel comfortable sharing our truths. Where we balance Tom's perspective and needs," as he said this Dr. Amare placed his hand on my left knee and looked me in the eyes before turning back to Doc, "with yours and vice versa. Today we will get to know each other better and at each subsequent visit more and more. Today we will begin to develop a relationship foundation in which to build and grow together on this healing journey. And today I will begin to understand each of your preferences," Dr. Amare paused for a moment and then, "and that starts right now with this conversation."

And with that, I noticed Doc nodding as Dr. Amare sat back and took another moment to look at both Doc and me … together.

"I have had a chance to review your quite hefty medical record, Tom. Thank you for sending it over prior to our visit today. And we will get to that for sure. For now, though I want to talk about the both of you."

And as we talked about our relationship, the way we support and depend on each other in different ways and so much more, I noticed Dr. Amare truly focusing on each of us.

I also noticed he had not placed a laptop between us nor turned away to face a computer of some sort. Rather he had found a balance of engaging with each of us, listening intently and feeding back to us what he has heard, (I assume to ensure accuracy), and occasionally handwriting a note or two.

This dynamic within the healthcare system felt incredibly foreign to me.

For the past few months, I had been referred to as a number, as a diagnosis, and as 'him' even when I was in the room. Dr. Amare continuously referred to Doc and me as Darlene and Tom.

Here, today, I saw Dr. Amare's eyes. His face. His smile.

Here today I felt cared for. And I felt my wife was being cared for too.

Already I felt the flame of hope, that Tory had helped to fan, growing just a little bit more.

And just about sixty minutes later …

"Wonderful. Darlene do you now see why it is so important that you are here today?"

"I do. We are a team."

Ah, my Brockton girl putting things into a sports analogy.

"And as a team, we need to be on the same page. We need to be supporting one another."

God, she is good, I thought and then verbalized, "and together we need to develop a game plan."

"Exactly. We are all in this together. We all have a role to play. This is not about me and what I want for you two. This is not about my plan for you, Tom. This is about you both, and your goals, your preferences, and how I can help support you in your journey to achieve these goals … according to those preferences."

Dr. Amare paused for a moment as he again sat back in his chair, "And today we have confirmed that you both want to engage fully in this process together. Correct?"

Interestingly both Doc and I simultaneously reached out for one another's hand, me with my left and her with her right, and held one another, "Oh yes."

"Wonderful. Now Tom, tell me about this flight to Seattle and what happened."

And for the next forty-five minutes, between bouts of coughing and taking deep breaths, I shared my story, with Doc adding pieces that I missed either because I was unaware or had simply forgotten.

Go Team! I thought each time she provided another nugget of wisdom that would have been lost without her present and in my corner. (Yes, another boxing reference. From Brockton, you know.)

We discussed the flight. And then with Dr. Amare's prompting, we discussed what led up to the flight.

"He was so stressed. He wasn't sleeping."

"Why, Tom? What was going on at that time?"

At this I remember hesitating and looking at the floor. It felt like a thousand thoughts were going through my head as I struggled to respond.

"Was this related to your home-life or your work or both or other stressors, Tom?"

Doc looked at me and saw I was deep in thought and struggling so she began to answer, "Dr. Amare, Tom was very stressed over many changes being made at work that he did not believe were best for his members and patients."

I continued from there.

"We care for folks who are military retirees and others who are the dependents of active duty military personnel. And after sharing time with these people, gaining understanding into the number of health challenges they face each day, the chronic illnesses they are battling, the mental health challenges, in addition to socio-economic realities," I was getting agitated, and I was sure it was coming through as I felt that all too familiar pressure on my chest and struggled to breathe. "I believed many decisions being made throughout the healthcare system would lead to harm… it was breaking my heart."

As I finished, Doc placed her hand on my shoulder as I felt my sweat seep through.

We continued on with this part of the discussion for quite some time.

And honestly, I was still taken aback at both the time we were sharing with Dr. Amare as well as the level of transparency and amount of information we were all providing.

"No way this level of sharing … this level of caring happens in a ten-minute office visit," I thought as my head began to pound again and my breath became more labored.

For the next part of our visit, we discussed my journey through the healthcare system associated with this illness to date. The medications, the procedures, all the physicians I had seen, the impact of all of the above and then Dr. Amare surprised me a bit…

"Tell me how you were feeling emotionally during this journey."

Not being used to having this type of discussion with a physician, I hesitated. Yes, we had shared a great deal of time together today, in fact probably more time together in this one visit than the total amount of time I had spent with any one physician I had seen over the past many months except for maybe my cardiologist and primary care physician. But still. Sharing emotions with a physician?

"I have felt like a failure."

Not sure why I said it, but I did.

"Oh Tom, you are not a failure in any sense of the word," Doc responded to me as she quickly took my hand again.

Momma Bear.

"Why Tom? Why have you felt like a failure?" Dr. Amare inquired.

And for the first time with my bride, and of course with Dr. Amare, I shared the story of my amazing team, the lessons we had learned, the course we had set together to make things better, (to counteract the brokenness of the healthcare system), and how my illness had taken me away from this and thus had let my team and all these people down.

"I failed," I said out loud.

And then as I watched Doc look at me with so much love, I continued, "And I have failed Doc and our children. I am supposed to take care of my family. I am supposed to provide. I am supposed to be able to play with my kids. I am supposed to not yell at them when they ask for cereal …."

At this, I re-entered my body (as Doc says) and felt all the recent pains ….

A pain from my left shoulder traveled through my neck and stabbed at my temple as a sledgehammer pounded again at my chest, just like back in the day at the Y when I missed the rack and dropped a barbell while benching.

My head was now in my hands as the tears rolled harshly down my cheeks and onto Dr. Amare's rug.

"Tom. … Tommy. No. No one thinks you are a failure. No one," Doc started and then she paused before continuing, "Listen to me. And listen good. No one thinks you are a failure. Your team doesn't. They love you. Your peers don't. They have reached out with so much care and love for you and our family. I certainly don't. And you know the kids love you."

She was hugging me now with our temples touching and our tears flowing together.

"And you know," Doc was smiling a little now as she reminded me, "Angus loves you, too."

As I sat with my love, I began to breathe again. Breathe in the energy of the two of us. Breathe in the release of finally saying out loud what I had been feeling so deeply for so long. And breathe in the words my bride was saying to me.

And then after what seemed like ten minutes of silence (except for my breathing) ….

"What else you got, Dr. Amare?" I said with a grin as I felt a wave of exhaustion run over me.

"Tom, you clearly have wonderful support from Darlene. And now I am on your team too. We have much work to do together and many emotions will be raised. And as they are, addressing them will be part of your healing journey."

Doc and I were still holding hands as Dr. Amare continued.

"There is physical healing and there is emotional healing. And I bet with each of your many sports injuries you have experienced many emotions that perhaps you did not address at that time. Would that be accurate?"

"Oh yes, Doctor. Even now he still tries to demonstrate he can still play ball like he is eighteen years old … I believe because he thinks he has something to prove."

Thanks, Doc. I thought as I also acknowledge both she and Dr. Amare were correct.

"So yes, physical healing, emotional healing (which is necessary relative to almost all illnesses and/or injuries), mental health healing (which in this context is the impact on your mental health when dealing with this acute illness and all of its impacts). All three of these aspects of health are very important."

I, of course, recognized the importance of the mental health aspect of healthcare, especially as of late relative to my military folks and seeing the mental health challenges they were facing … and how we were letting them down.

Throughout the healthcare system we were not only focusing on increasing revenue production via shorter visits (and thus ensuring limited time for the mental health aspect of care to be even mentioned never mind addressed and coordinated), but we were also turfing mental healthcare to an outside vendor as if it was totally separate from the physical health of our patients. Like we could split a patient and say "Bring your diabetes health issues to this doctor and your mental health challenges to that doctor across town. And don't worry, there is no connection between the two."

Oh yes, on this I was right in line with Dr. Amare's thinking. I just naively didn't expect it to include me.

"That makes great sense, Doctor," Doc said, as I nodded my head while still in deep thought.

And together for the next fifteen minutes, the three of us began the discussion of my illness and its impact on my mental health as well as the mental health of Doc and the kids. Again, all foreign territory for Doc and me.

"Now let's talk about spiritual health. We have talked about physical, emotional, and mental health. Tell me about your spiritual beliefs."

My god, what kind of doctor is this? I thought as I also wondered if Doc is thinking the same thing. *My spiritual beliefs? Really? How do I answer that?*

But I figured, we had come this far, I already felt like I had been on an emotional rollercoaster … *might as well play until the whistle.*

"We were both brought up Catholic and continue to practice our Faith," I began. "I was also an altar boy and boy scout in my youth. Our, or I will simply say 'my' (so that Doc can respond for herself), my faith is very important to me. I pray every day for guidance and strength. And on occasion battle it out as to His will or mine. Clearly a losing proposition."

"And I feel the same way (even the battle aspect)," Doc added.

"Clearly God has been yelled at quite a bit by members of the Dahlborg household over the last several months."

We talked with Dr. Amare more about our spiritual beliefs and also asked him about his. It was a fascinating discussion which reminded me of those times sitting around the camp table in Maine after snowmobiling with my cousins and hearing them talk about their strong faith. Powerful, to say the least.

And then we came to the time when we needed to wrap up.

"Darlene, I don't know if Tom will ever work again," Dr. Amare said in response to Doc. And then he looked at both of us and said, "But I do know this. Together we will create a care pathway which will best position you to do so, Tom. We will schedule our second appointment for tomorrow and then from there we will schedule check-ins either in person, via Email, or by phone at least every three days to ensure the path we have chosen continues to be the right one. And if not, together we will modify the plan." And then looking first at Doc, then at me, and then at both of us, "How does that sound to you both?"

Both Doc and I were clearly exhausted from the intensity of the time we had just shared with Dr. Amare. But I believe we both felt relief in hearing that we were in this together, and we would be checking in so often.

"It sounds great," I said as clearly as I could as I struggled for breath.

"It really does, Dr. Amare."

"Wonderful. And one last thing, now that we have gotten to know each other a bit, please, if you are comfortable, please simply call me Ben."

REFLECTION

Some time ago I was astounded to find quite a bit of "woo woo" language in the Hippocratic Oath that suggests empathy is part of true healing.

For example, the Oath says:

> *"I will remember that there is art to medicine as well as science, and that warmth, sympathy, and understanding may outweigh the surgeon's knife or the chemist's drug."*

Who would have thought that warmth and sympathy could potentially be more important than the surgeon's knife or a prescription drug in healing?

Considering the myriad reimbursement models emphasizing production and invasive procedures (rather than time to develop relationships and trust) and the priority given to drug therapies, our current healthcare "system", does not believe this to be the case.

Another example:

> *"I will remember that I do not treat a fever chart, a cancerous growth, but a sick human being, whose illness may affect the person's family and economic stability. My responsibility includes these related problems, if I am to care adequately for the sick."*

Could there possibly be holism, or taking all of a patient's physical, mental and social conditions into account during the health encounter, in the Hippocratic Oath? Could it be that episodic and siloed intervention-based care is not the way to truly position individuals, families, and communities for better health?

To date, most existing physician practices, hospitals, physician hospital organizations (PHOs), as well as newer "innovations" in healing such as patient-centered medical homes (PCMHs) and accountable care organizations (ACOs) are not truly embracing holism in healing. They are not designed to focus on the patient as a whole person along with the family system and the economic impact to the family due to a specific health crisis. These existing organizations and "innovations" do not currently nor intend to integrate the physical, mental, environmental and financial drivers impacting patients, families and communities. Apparently holistic care, which according to the Hippocratic Oath focuses on the person (not the disease), is still "woo woo" in the eyes of our staid medical system.

Again, based on current and proposed reimbursement models (where only small portions of revenue are tied to outcomes via Pay for Performance (P4P) models), short office visits, a lack of true integration of even mental health with primary care (never mind social and economic factors), and rotating practitioners and extenders, it appears that in fact holism is not part of the current healthcare "system" nor future "innovations." And yet ... it is very clearly part of the Hippocratic Oath physicians pledge to honor.

Here's a third example:

> *"May I always act so as to preserve the finest traditions of my calling and may I long experience the joy of healing those who seek my help."*

> *"The joy of healing?" (Have you talked with a physician recently?)*

Whatever happened to "joy in healing"? Neither the current system nor the new "innovations" are set up to truly focus on the health and satisfaction (the joy) of the physician (the healer). The design is still based on maximizing financial return on investment and productivity, not maximizing health status improvement and physician satisfaction. And just try to discuss "the joy of healing" in most healthcare organizations and watch out. ... Be prepared for laughter, scorn, and being marginalized as a healer.

Hippocrates and the subsequent evolution of the Hippocratic Oath truly understood healing. Call it "woo woo," call it squishy, call it warm and fuzzy ... call it what you will. But as the Oath illustrates, warmth, sympathy, understanding, holism and joy in healing are critical factors required for any optimal healing model.

Questions

1. As a clinician, how often do you discuss the emotional, the mental, and the spiritual aspects of health and healing with your patient?

2. There are many forms of spirituality and/or religious practice; and yet not everyone has a spiritual practice. As a patient, have your spiritual beliefs been embraced and honored as you have engaged the healthcare system either as a patient, family member, or as a clinician?

3. What recommendations would you make to improve this practice?

Chapter 45

Rest My Love

Sleep the previous evening remained a trial. Between the headache and shoulder pain, the chest pressure and chest pain, and the constant dry cough getting more than an hour of sleep at a time remained a rare blessing.

Doc said she slept okay but, knowing her the way I do, I was sure she was also up stressing about me as we continued to sleep apart.

The vividness of my many dreams and nightmares remained as well. One would think with such limited sleep they would dissipate. Well, one would be wrong.

From escaping the depths of oblivion to soaring into the light of day; from sea creatures burrowing through my body to opening my eyes to an Irish angel looking upon me with grace and love; and from suffocating from the weight of the dark and unknown to escaping into a bright castle in the sky, the many dreams kept the night interesting to say the least.

At least they tend to end positively now as opposed to me screaming into the night, I thought as I looked back at the past several months.

"How did you sleep?"

Ah yes, the same question each morning. *God, how I miss sleeping with my bride,* I thought as I tried to be creative in my response.

Oh well, nothing witty this morning so, "I slept okay. Missed you. Angus cuddled a bit but nothing like you."

"I missed you too. Every night I miss you holding me."

It is an amazing thing to experience a partnership flourish. In business for sure but also in a marriage. It is even better to be a part of the partnership. In our case, noting it was not always easy by any means, we continued to grow and evolve in our marriage, in our love for one another, and in our partnership. Of course, my illness had been an incredible test for us, and it was truly hard and yet ... and yet we had found a way so far.

There were some days when we were both strong. And while we supported one another, we were also able to focus on each of our own paths and continue to move forward.

On other days, only one of us was able to be strong. I know there had been many days where either my ego, or my fear, or my disappointment led me down some very dark paths. And it was on those days Doc would say, "Tom, I love you, you don't need to be strong for us at this moment. I will be strong for us both right now. It is my turn."

And even though I would perhaps go down an even darker path as I thought about how I MUST be strong, I would also know (or come to realize) that she was right. We were partners and at this specific time, her role was to be the strong one.

And at other times, like on this morning, I would sense that Doc was tired, and I needed to be strong for both of us. It was our deal. It was our marriage. It was our love. And it was our partnership.

Rest, my love. I have got this. I will get better, and I will come back to you stronger and wiser than I had ever been. I love you beyond my words or my broken heart. You will be safe in my arms. Now and always.

Slowly I raised myself off of the couch and made my way over to Doc as she peered out the kitchen window into our side yard and took her first sip of coffee. As I approached, I again noticed the moistness of her gorgeous blue eyes.

Then from behind I slipped my arms around her waist and whispered, "You are so strong for me and the kids. You have been holding us all together for so long. Today is my day to hold you, my love. It is my turn."

Doc didn't say anything as her shoulders lowered just a bit and she leaned back into my chest and let the back of her head nestle under my chin.

"I've got you today. I've got you," I whispered over and over as I held the love of my life for an eternity. *Yes*, I thought, *holding my bride for eternity. God, this is all I want.*

As Doc and I drove to my second appointment with Dr. Amare, we continued to process the events from our first visit.

"Even though at first it felt awkward, I liked being so engaged with you and Ben as part of your healing process. How did it feel for you having me there?"

"I wouldn't say it felt awkward." And then with a smile, I added with great emphasis on the word 'always', "You know I *always* love being with you." And we both laughed.

"Seriously though, I didn't find it awkward. More so, like you said yesterday, I felt like we were creating a team. A care team. But different than a typical care team."

"Darlene, Tom, welcome back."

Dr. Amare had emerged from his office and was now walking toward Doc and me. He was wearing brown slacks, a tan shirt with no tie, and casual brown shoes. He also had a big smile on his face as he approached us once again with his hand extended.

"Good morning, Dr. Amare."

"Come on in. Come on in."

"I have looked over your medical record in depth. You have quite a history of injuries and a good number of surgeries."

For the next 45 minutes or so we discussed each of these injuries, how they occurred, how I felt, the decision process to elect to have the surgery or not, the specific type of surgery, and the outcome.

"Now tell me more about these headaches you are having?"

Then for the next 25 minutes or so we discussed my headaches. The possible connection to the shoulder injury, my long-term use of Naproxen to manage the pain, and the switch to Vioxx. In addition to again the emotional toll of the pain, and even the impact from a mental perspective as more and more I was restricted in what I could do.

We also discussed how I engaged spiritually in my process to live with and manage the pain.

And I was again astounded at our connection and sharing.

I also noted my feelings of gratitude in having Doc share insights that I was not necessarily aware of, "I notice that whenever he does anything over his head, light or heavy, be it painting a ceiling or fixing a light bulb, he will be in intense pain that evening due to the pain in his shoulder, neck and head. Every time. And he won't be able to sleep."

It was wonderful to learn and share with Doc and with Ben in this way. I truly did feel we were becoming that care team we all wanted.

And I remember thinking that this process was also cathartic for Doc as she got to hear and see me in a whole different way … vulnerable. Which, quite frankly, was not easy at all. Especially this early in this new setting.

She heard a lot of what I typically processed in my mind. She heard me confess the emotional toll all of this was taking on me. She heard the details of the pain I had been feeling (and which I had tried to hide). She saw me weak and afraid.

And this was so hard. So very hard.

But as we continued this sharing, I knew I needed to "gut it out" and surrender to this vulnerability if I was to prevail and get healthy again.

Courage through vulnerability.

And I got to see Doc also share much I was unaware of. Her pains and fears.

> "I don't want to lose my husband."

> "I am so scared and feel so alone."

> "What would Tommy do without a dad? Sammy? Haylee?"

> "I cry myself to sleep."

Yes, I got to see her heart and soul. And it was hard.

And yes, we manifested our partnership in a whole new way. And in partnership with Ben.

"I have a good picture of what is going on with that head pain. And I am not enamored with your need to rely on either Naproxen or Vioxx. So let's get you relieved of this pain, off of these meds, and some much needed rest. What do you say?"

Relief from constant pain even when I am not taking an NSAID or COX-2 inhibitor? Rest? Sleep? I am all in, I thought.

"But doctor, when Tom misses even one dose of Naproxen or Vioxx now he suffers so."

God, I love her.

"We are going to change that. We are going to get Tom some rest. And when you come back, we will focus directly on Tom's heart."

Of course, I was thrilled to hear the confidence married to the caring in Ben's voice. While interestingly at the same time I kept thinking, "But will insurance pay for all of this time together?"

For our remaining time this day, the three of us co-created a treatment plan specific to me, my injuries, my history, my goals and my preferences in order to relieve my shoulder, neck and head pain with an aim of providing me with an opportunity to truly rest and position me to heal my heart.

"Do you both understand the next steps? What to do? What to look for?"

"Yes," Doc and I responded in unison.

"Excellent. Together we will adjust this plan as necessary. No worries. Now the both of you, go home and rest. Take care of one another. And I will see you back here tomorrow."

REFLECTION

When health systems say 'care teams,' it is typically defined as a patient and his or her doctor, plus a physician assistant and/or a nurse practitioner, a nurse, a medical assistant, or more.

Some practices truly leverage these team members to improve the care and safety for patients. Others, however, use these teams to increase productivity and revenue generation while decreasing overhead ... rather than improve care.

The team approach may provide some benefits, be it financial or other, but it is at the expense of the continuity between a patient and 'their' doctor, which I heard loud and clear through our focus groups and voice of the customer processes; as well as years later as part a number of quality improvement and research-related engagements.

An unintended consequence of care teams is the fact that many patients will not feel a bond with the ever-changing clinician, will not share their whole story or that nugget of insight and wisdom that could be leveraged to help keep them safe and better positioned on their care journey.

Patients want to see their own doctor or their nurse. They want to have an authentic relationship with a (with their) trusted clinician. They don't want to see a different person at each visit. They don't want to have to tell their story over and over again to each new clinician.

Patients want to feel cared for and about. And interestingly so do doctors and nurses.

It is on us healthcare leaders to innovate and develop a model that meets this aim.

Questions

1. As a patient, do you feel you have a doctor and/or nurse who truly cares about you?

2. As a clinician, do you truly know each of your patients? Do you truly care about them?

3. As a patient, do you trust the clinician you see?

    a. Do you share key insights you have into your care journey?

    b. If not, what prevents you from doing so?

4. As a clinician, do you trust your patients?

    a. Do you believe they share all pertinent information with you?

    b. If not, what do you believe prevents them from doing so?

5. What recommendations would you make to ensure optimal authentic connection and sharing between patients and clinicians?

Chapter 46

A New Model

Visit three with Dr. Amare began as per usual. A warm greeting from Mary. A just as warm greeting from Ben. And an invitation to join him in his office.

Doc and I again sat side by side and Ben again sat in front of us.

And again, there was nothing between us. No PC. No laptop. No desk. We were all joined together in a common space. In what was becoming more and more our safe space.

A safe space where my care team, the care team comprised of my family, my doctor, and I, could co-create care plans that garnered wisdom from each of us. Doc's nursing background and wisdom plus her knowledge of me and our eleven years together, and her huge heart, combined with all I know and feel and can contribute, combined with Ben's medical wisdom and his caring was a powerful combination.

And when we add that we were each developing a deeper and more authentic relationship in which a trust that I had never experienced with a caregiver could blossom … we knew we truly had something.

A new medical model, I remember thinking. *A medical model that focused on the physical, mental, emotional, and spiritual aspects of health and healing (and dying for those on that journey) in conjunction with the latest evidence-based medicine, a physician who is whole and healthy him or herself, families engaged, and all stakeholders having the time to truly connect in an authentic way. This is how medicine should be. This is what my members and patients want.*

And then thinking further, *This is probably how medicine was back in the day. At least the components of what I am seeing and experiencing as compassion, empathy, relationship, trust, and the four-dimensional focus of physical, mental, emotional, and spiritual health. Imagine marrying this with cutting-edge technology tools, pharmaceuticals, latest evidenced-based medicine based on reliable research outcomes, and joy in healing for doctors and nurses? Hmmmm … isn't that from the Hippocratic Oath?*

I paused as Doc and Ben turned to me to ask for my input and then continued my thinking, *Perhaps this is truly what Ben has created. Or at least parts of it.*

"Tom. Where are you right now? Clearly you are not here with us."

"I am sorry, Ben. I was just thinking about your practice and how in just three visits, we have come further in our relationship as doctor and patient and family then I have ever done before with any physician. And how even though this is wicked hard," yes, a little bit of my Brockton (or some would say Boston) came through, "and yet our process feels right."

"I see," and then before he could finish …

"Ben, this is one of the challenges I believe Tom creates for himself. I want him to focus on his healing, but his mind never stops."

Doc was beginning to tear up again now.

"I just want him to come back to me healthy again. Right now, I want him to focus on his own healing." And then turning to me, "We talked about this. You need to focus on you right now."

The three of us discussed this further. Not because it was a challenging topic (which it was) but more so because we were exploring this from many angles. We didn't arrive at a particular answer and yet, we each shared from both our hearts and minds, Doc and I each cried a bit, and we each felt better having gotten this out in the open.

Then after another dry coughing spell and an opportunity to get some water, we continued with a keen focus on my heart.

"I really don't know if you will ever get back to work," Ben said again while looking directly at me and in response to my question.

But rather than go to a dark place, I remember making note that to have an authentic relationship it must include transparency and discussing the hard stuff. Not hiding or avoiding it. It means dealing with conflict appropriately not hiding from it.

"But through our work together, we now have a care path that will provide you," Ben continued to focus directly on me, "the best opportunity to do so. And as part of the implementation of this plan, we are going to do the following: We are going to check in at least every three days via office visits. In the meantime, you will contact me by phone or E-mail with any questions, concerns, significant changes, fears, happy thoughts … anything and at any time. Do you understand?"

"Yes, I do," I responded while also thinking I was not going to call Ben at 3:00am with a 'happy thought.'

"And for each three-day cycle, I will share with you what I believe the three paths that your healing journey will take and what to do on each path. As an example, for the next three days I predict one of three things will happen: 1.) …"

And Ben shared his prediction. He said if his first prediction came true, even though painful and scary, it is expected and I should do the following … which he described in detail. He then shared his second prediction and here, too, he provided Doc and me with a game plan to follow. And lastly, he shared his third prediction, which again he described in detail and made note that if this was to happen to immediately call an ambulance and get to the hospital.

He then let us know if anything other than these three things were to occur, we were to contact him immediately and together we would determine our next steps. That said, he also reassured us that at any point if we thought something was wrong, we could immediately call an ambulance. And then to contact him after we were sure I was safe.

A game plan that we created together. Check-ins at least every three days. Predictions and treatment plans for each eventuality. Options at our discretion. Continuity and availability of a doctor who engages my wife in my treatment and who clearly cares about me. Even though I was still in great discomfort and quite frankly petrified … I felt better.

By day two of the three-day window between office visits Ben's first prediction came true. And he was right, I was in intense pain, and it was scary. And yet, this was expected and we were prepared.

"Tom, do you want to go the Emergency Room?"

My visceral reaction was, "My chest and my head are going to explode. Call the ambulance!" But we had our plan and as I tried to visualize and breathe through the pain as my mom had taught me, I also remembered Ben's prediction.

"Not yet, Doc. Not yet. I just want to somehow get some sleep. To sleep through this."

"Then let's call Ben. He said to do so if we have any concerns. And you are clearly in so much pain."

In three visits we had come so very far. And yet relationship and trust takes time to develop. We were getting there but …

"Doc, Ben predicted this. In fact, this was his first prediction. We have a plan for this. But, yes, let's call him to make sure. I think that is the prudent thing to do."

(I am actually not sure if I said prudent at the time but thinking back it was what I meant.)

"Dr. Amare, this is Darlene Dahlborg. Tom is in so much pain. He …"

Doc explained to Ben my situation over the phone. She asked me specific questions as per Ben's requests and ten minutes later …

"Tom, Ben was glad we called. We are on the right path. He said at any point we can still get you to the hospital but that he expected you to feel this way by today. And that like he said it is actually a good thing. A sign we are on the right path."

Doc continued to share and even just hearing this reassurance from Ben and Doc, I felt better.

"Do you want to go to the hospital just in case, my love?"

"No, Honey." Oops. "We have our plan. We are on it. If, like you said after talking with Ben, things get worse, then yes. But for now, let's stay the course."

And that is what we did and by day three I was feeling a little better and on my way back to see Dr. Amare for the fourth time.

"Darlene, Tom, great to see you. Come on in. Come on in."

"Great to see you too, Dr. Amare."

It was still not easy for Doc or me to call Dr. Amare by his first name, Ben. So, on occasion he was Ben and at other times he was Dr. Amare.

"Let's discuss these past three days. Tell me …"

And for the next 90 minutes the three of us, my care team, discussed the multi-dimensions of my health (and also of Doc's health as my caregiver).

We discussed what happened on day two. How we felt from all four dimensions. And what we did. Ben reviewed my medical record with us, we again discussed my latest test results, and we discussed how we both were today.

And again, and together, we set a three-day course of action with predictions, options, contingencies, assurances, and next steps.

And then we left Ben's office with a plan. Our plan.

For the next few weeks and then eventually the next few months, my care team connected at least every three days to review my care plan, to assess its multi-dimensional impact, and to modify our course as necessary based on outcomes, our collective wisdom and trust for one another.

"Tom, we are four weeks together, we believe there has been great progress with your head, neck and shoulder, and based on your goals we have set together, I believe it is time to stop taking the Vioxx."

The three of us had set (and then reset) a number of goals for me, with of course the most important being focused on my heart. Positioning me to sleep better by eliminating the pain in my head was part of the plan.

"When you stop the Vioxx I predict one of three things will happen. If this ..."

Again, Ben walked Doc and me through his predictions and provided us with specific next steps, options, and a contingency plan. We were now accustomed to this routine and yet still amazed that healthcare in 2001 could be so relationship-focused and caring with an emphasis on shared decision making based on our mutual trust, whole story, and openness.

And, yes, to answer my earlier question, my insurance was paying for these visits and this approach to care. Which I was still having trouble believing. *It can be done*, I said to myself as I also thought about the savings to the system if, in fact, I can get to the point where I no longer need to take daily meds.

Going from the expectation and the expense of taking a pill every day for the rest of my life to possibly stopping altogether was surreal. Better care, better outcomes, better experience, reduced costs.

It can be done, I thought as I began to get excited again and I turned to the Almighty, "My GOD ... if I do get well, perhaps Your Will is okay after all. Perhaps I am meant to help change the system with this new knowledge based on my real-life experience. Perhaps..."

And then I caught myself as Doc's words flowed into my mind, "Tom, focus on your healing first. You can only help others when you are well."

"Now let's turn our attention back to your heart, Tom. And this time let's focus first on the mental health aspect of your healing."

I loved that Ben constantly spoke of 'healing.'

And again, we spent forty-five minutes or so discussing the mental, physical, emotional and spiritual dimensions associated with my diagnosis of viral myocarditis. I again shared my continuing fear of leaving my wife and kids, of causing them so much stress and pain, and of letting my team and those we serve down as I did it.

I shared my physical symptoms and how each day I am noticing a number of changes. Some good. Some not so much. The chest pressure and pain. The dry coughing spells. The difficulty breathing. The fatigue.

I shared how I yell at God when I get desperate. How mad I get. How I hate not having control and how I hate God's Will if it is different from mine.

I cried as I again shared my many failures in so many areas and especially how I am now a burden to my wife and kids.

It was so hard. Even in this safe space, it was so hard to continue to admit out loud. And as I did, my breaths got shorter and shorter and my coughing got worse.

And as I went on and on, Ben nodded his head. He asked clarifying questions. He handed me a box of tissues.

He truly listened.

He truly understood.

He truly cared.

As did Doc. My beautiful, caring, loving, tough bride … she listened, she understood, she cared. Like she always does.

Now I wish I could say I felt better with all this sharing.

But no. Rather, I shared because I believed in Ben and our process. I believed that the best chance for me to get well was to follow this path. And for my wife and children, and for my team, and for all those I cared about I was willing to be vulnerable in this way because I believed if I remained true to the process then I would get closer to regaining my health and making things up to all these people I cherish and love.

So, no. While this sharing was important and I knew I was in a safe place, it still was hard. It still impacted my ego and hurt my soul.

"Okay, Darlene, Tom, do you understand the plan for the next three days? Tom, do you understand what to do relative to your shoulder, neck, and head pain? Do you understand what to do relative to your heart? And you will call me immediately with any questions or concerns?"

Being four weeks in and having co-created our plan, Doc and I answered affirmatively to each of these questions.

"Wonderful. And Tom, I am not going to tell you not to worry. I will simply say, you are showing great courage in your sharing and your honesty, in your focus, and in your ability to face so much pain at one time. I want you to hold that close when you feel anxious or down. I want you to focus on your ability to be courageous in your vulnerability. That, right now, is a flame burning bright within your soul."

"Thank you, Ben," was all I could say as we left his office and then the building.

I didn't feel courageous. I felt like I was simply following our plan.

Three days later …

"Ben, I stopped taking the Vioxx the day after we last met. It petrified me because I know how intense the pain can get."

"Ben, I hate hearing Tom pace all night due to that pain. Or him on all fours with his head buried in his pillow as he rocks back and forth all night because of it. So honestly, I too, was scared for him to stop the meds."

I hadn't known Doc could hear me pacing all those times. I knew she knew about the rocking because I would be right next to her in bed back in the day. But the pacing, I had thought I was Batman.

"And how are you feeling?" Ben asked us both.

"I am almost afraid to say, but so far I have had no pain in my shoulder, neck or head, since stopping. I believe the care plan we put together for me is really working."

"And you, Darlene?"

"Oh Ben, any relief for Tommy …"

Tommy? I remember thinking.

"… I just want him out of as much pain as possible. I am so happy."

As I reached over to put my arm around Doc, I could see tears in her eyes again.

"I just want this to last. Will it, Doctor?" Doc asked as I held her.

"I believe the path we created is the right one. We will keep monitoring and adjust as necessary," responded Ben.

Another six days later …

"Ten days without Vioxx and without pain in your shoulder, neck and head. Excellent. Now tell me about your breathing."

"My breathing is better. And I have been making it upstairs to sleep in our bed again."

I hadn't been upstairs since God and I had an epic battle months and months ago over whose Will we were going to follow. Needless to say, I lost that battle.

"I am not saying if that is a good or bad thing," Doc added as she smiled and shared her beautiful distinctive laugh.

Doc is joking, I thought with great joy. *I am the butt of her joke, but she is joking.*

And we all laughed.

Three more days later …

"Still no pain in your shoulder, neck, and head. Excellent. And your breathing continues to improve."

"Yes, as I said I was able to walk up and down the street with Doc this week."

"Excellent. Tell me how you are feeling emotionally."

Another six days later …

"We have made progress with your shoulder, neck and head pain. You are now walking consistently. We have modified your treatment plan a few times. Your dry cough has subsided greatly. Tell me about the pain and pressure on your chest."

As usual Ben had reviewed our plan, my treatments, the modifications we had made, and the outcomes. And with this information at hand we discussed the most recent impact of each.

"Each day it seems as though it lessens more and more. I now go up and down the stairs a few times a day with less chest pain and pressure. I am walking as you noted. The pain is much less but does exacerbate when I get stressed …"

"Ben, Tom's pain worsens when he gets stressed either physically or mentally. Right, honey?"

Of course, I wanted to say *don't honey me*, but I didn't.

"Yes, that is true Ben. Will that change?"

"I believe as you continue to heal, yes, that will change. It will lessen as you get stronger. But it will take time."

"I know. I know. But we have come so far. And I am feeling so much better. I guess I just want it all now."

"I tell him 'have patience,' Ben."

"Listen to Darlene, Tom. She knows." Ben said with a big smile.

And after another shared laugh, I added …

"Ben, I still get that sense of impending doom. Is that normal?"

"Tell me more."

Another twenty-four days later …

"Ben, I remain off of the Vioxx and the NSAIDs and still have very limited if any pain in my shoulder, neck and head. I am sleeping through the night most of the time. The pressure and pain in my chest is much better and only noticeable when I am stressed and tired. I want the greenlight to go back to work. I want to make a difference again. I no longer want to be a burden to Doc and the kids. Please, give me the green light."

"Darlene, what are you thinking?"

"Oh Ben, Tom's health is so much better. He is running (sort of) around with the kids, playing on the floor, giving them horsey and piggy-back rides. And quite frankly," here comes her smile and laugh again, "He is becoming a pain in the butt around the house. Let him go back to work!"

We all start laughing, and I unfortunately start coughing that dry cough of mine.

No, I think as I try to hold it back. *Not now. I want to go to work!*

We all talked a great deal more. And, as always, we focused on the physical, mental, emotional, and spiritual dimensions of my and Doc's health. We reviewed our co-created treatment plan (and its many modifications over time) and interventions to date. What worked and what didn't. What exacerbates my symptoms and what helps. We reviewed the latest test results. We discussed the next three days and the next three after that and the next three after that. We reviewed predictions.

Ben then circled back to my emotional health, "Tom, tell me more about why you want to go back to work now."

I remember at this point taking another breath as I was beginning to get emotional again.

"Ben, I am ready to go back. I know that I am no longer the COO, and I am not even sure if Saul will take me back…"

"Of course he will, Tom," Doc whispered as she placed her right hand on my left knee.

"... well, if he does Ben, I feel like I may be able to do some good."

We talked for another ten or fifteen minutes.

And then Ben said, "Tom, I do believe you are ready to go back. Part-time to start. And as you do, we will continue our work together, we will continue to follow our path, we will continue to check in, and we will continue to adjust. How does that sound?"

REFLECTION

Carl was a funeral home director in Brockton for many years, and one of those lesser known legends. In fact, what became known as Dahlborg-MacNevin Funeral Home is a pseudo landmark for many in Brockton.

Now some might find being a funeral home director creepy or eerie or morbid, but not me. Because this funeral home director was my Grandpa.

When I was young, my father used to take me to Bob the Barber for my haircut. This was back when you didn't call ahead for an appointment but rather would simply show up, sit in a smoke-filled room with a bunch of other guys, read comic books, listen to the adults talk about the Red Sox and how Lou Gorman made another terrible trade but how next year was going to be our year, and wait your turn.

I actually loved going to see Bob. But not for any of the above. Rather, because Bob had been around forever (at least it seemed that way to me), grew up with my parents, and knew everybody. But most important to me, he knew my Grandpa.

"Oh yes, Tommy. Your grandfather would come in for his haircut all dressed in his black suit. He would sit and talk sports and politics with the guys and laugh politely at our silly jokes. But it was funny how the guys thought he was a minister. So as soon as they saw him, all the swearing would stop."

I so loved hearing about Grandpa.

"Tommy, back in the day, many people in town were very poor. The shoe industry was not always doing well, and people would be finding it very hard to pay their bills. And when there was a death in the family of one of these poor people, who was the person who would take care of everything for them and not charge a dime? It was your grandfather. Yes, it was Carl Dahlborg. A death on Christmas Eve, your grandfather would be sure to do whatever the family of the deceased needed him to do. 3am? No problem. Carl would be there comforting the family and making sure all was taking care of. Your Grandfather is a gentle man, Tommy. And he is a special man. You should be very proud."

Sitting and listening to Bob the Barber tell me about my Grandpa meant so much to me and only years later did the many levels of meaning begin to pop through.

Here was Bob, who was what one would call back in the day, "a man's man", tall, dark, handsome, athlete, entrepreneur, business owner, husband, father, telling me that my grandfather was special because he was caring. Here was Bob, someone I looked up to, sharing stories with me of my grandfather's compassion. Here was someone close to me telling me he admired my grandfather for so many reasons including that my grandfather was a gentle man.

Tom, I thought to myself many years later, it is okay to show that you care. It is okay to be compassionate. It is okay to be gentle. You can garner the respect of a Brocktonian and still be a gentle man. You don't have to hide your heart in business, in healthcare, in life.

Compassion, kindness, empathy and gentleness show strength (not weakness) ... and more importantly each better positions all of us to connect, to love, and to heal.

Questions

1. Who were/are your biggest influencers?
2. What have they taught you?
3. How have you manifested and honored this learning?
4. Do you feel you make them proud?
5. Please share a story of how you honor those you have learned from.

Chapter 47

A Second Chance

"Saul, its Tom. I would like to schedule a meeting with you to come in and discuss my future."

A few days later I was preparing to meet with Saul for the first time since I resigned.

"Doc, Saul has treated me so well. And now I am asking for him to create a position for me?"

After I resigned, rightfully so, Saul went out and hired a new COO for the military program. As I said, it was the right thing to do, I did resign, but nonetheless it still hurt deeply.

To know that under other circumstances I would still be in that seat leading my amazing team and positively impacting all those we serve, and especially our military folks … my heart truly hurt as I now sought another opportunity to be of service in a way that currently does not exist.

"Tom, you almost gave your life for them …"

A bit melodramatic I thought.

"… they will open their arms for you. To have you back and leading again, it only makes sense. Don't worry. Just talk to Saul. And whatever happens, happens. We will make do."

God she is good.

"Daddy, can you read to me?"

"Yes, Haylee. Of course. Climb up on my lap and I will read …"

Honestly, I have no idea what we read together. All I remember is holding my darling baby girl as I both read to her and thought about the next day.

Clearly not ideal parenting, and I told myself that, as I tried to be 100% present with my girl but was unsuccessful.

"Thank you, Daddy. I love sitting with you and reading our books."

"I do too, my love. I do too."

"Can we read another book together tomorrow, Daddy?"

Tomorrow? I thought. *Not too long ago I wasn't sure if I would have tomorrows with my children. And here I am already not 100% focused on my daughter. What is wrong with me?*

Over the next couple of hours, I, of course, rationalized my thinking and made every excuse for myself. But in the end, I knew there was no adequate rationalization. And I knew that I needed a HEARTchange … just like the system does… and right now. There was no waiting.

"Haylee!" I called upstairs believing she was now playing in her room. "Can we read another book together tonight? I would really like that."

And down from above came the voice of an angel, "Oh yes, Daddy. Yes. Let's read my 'Barney' book."

"Good morning, Saul."

"Tom, come on in. Come on in. How are you feeling?"

After some light banter, neither of our favorites I believe, I brought Saul up to speed on my health and the greenlight to return to work.

I also shared how grateful I was for him and the organization for all they had done for me and my family over these very long months. And how excited I was to serve again.

Mentioning I was "ready to serve again" was the hard part. Now that I was well, and at the same time someone else was sitting in my chair, I had no idea if I would be welcomed back. I also didn't know if there was funding for me. Or if there was even a position. Would the organization want to deal with a part-time, wounded employee? And if any of the above was a yes, would it be just out of pity? Would it be because they felt sorry for me?

The night before Doc and I had discussed 'pity' and how she believed the organization would want me back because they know me and that I have already proven my value. Not out of pity.

And she added, "They would be out of their minds not to."

And as we snuggled in bed under the warmth of the blankets, I confided in Doc that if they took me back out of pity it would absolutely "break my heart" but I would do it anyway for our family.

"Don't worry, Honey. Don't worry. God has a plan. No matter what Saul says tomorrow, there is a plan."

"Well, Tom, as you know after you resigned we went through a recruiting process and hired a new COO."

This isn't starting good, I thought as my chest grew heavy and my stomach hollowed.

"But," Saul began to continue.

Please God. Please, I prayed.

"Tom, I want to implement Hoshin planning across all three of our divisions."

And? I thought, *And?*

"I know you have been through the CQM training."

Could Saul be looking to me? My mind was already firing on all cylinders.

"We need focus, Tom. We need clarity. We need all of our divisions aligned and driving performance."

So far so good, I thought. *Focus, collaboration, alignment. Yes! I want in!*

"I want every person throughout the organization to know how they contribute to us achieving our Mission. And I want our mission achieved. I was about to begin a recruiting process to bring someone in for a year to drive this…"

What are you saying, Saul? What are you saying?

"This is not a C-level position, Tom, but the person in this role will have the opportunity to contribute to success in all of our divisions."

Is he selling me?

My heart was pounding. The pressure in my chest felt worse. I wanted to vomit. I had dreamed of this. I had hoped.

I want to pay my family and my team back. I want to help our members and patients. I want to bring all I learned over the past several months here so that I can help. *I don't care about title. I want to serve!* I thought as I realized I was losing track of what Saul was saying as a reluctant excitement grew inside of me.

"Tom, do you think you could handle this high-visibility, high-pressure role? Would you want this type of role? Because if you do …"

Please God. Please! I prayed as I also reminded myself, *Breathe Tom. Breathe.*

"… I would like to see you in it."

My God! My God! YES! YES! YES! THANK YOU! THANK YOU! THANK YOU! I want this so bad! I am going back to work! YES! YES! YES!

But, of course, I couldn't say all of that out loud. I needed to be professional.

"Wow, Saul. This sounds like a terrific role. Is there a job description? Who would this person be reporting to? What are the short-medium-long term goals?"

I have no idea where those words were coming from. In fact, I felt like I was outside of my body again watching someone else begin to negotiate a new job.

Thank you, God! I kept praying as Saul responded thoughtfully to each of my questions.

And after he had answered them all and we discussed a potential start I said, "Thank you, Saul. This opportunity is amazing. A chance to come back, be of service, and impact the entire organization … really amazing. If it will be alright with you, I will review the job description and discuss this with my bride this evening and let you know my final answer tomorrow."

I had no idea how I was remaining calm.

"Of course, Tom. I wouldn't want anything else. Go home, talk to Darlene, and call me tomorrow morning. And just so you know, I think you will do very well in this role."

I nearly floated out the front door of the administrative building.

Doc was waiting for me in the parking lot and by the time I reached her tears were streaming down my face.

"Oh Tom, what's the matter? What's the matter?"

At first, I couldn't respond. All my fears, all the darkness, all the pain, all the fatigue, all the sacrifices my wife and children had made, all the hard work, all the goodness, all the love … all the emotions attached to it all just started pouring out of me as I sat next to my bride and looked out onto Casco Bay.

I am going back to work, I thought as I sobbed.

"Tom. Tom. Tell me what's going on. We can figure whatever it is out. Just tell me."

Doc was being so patient as my mind was exploding with emotions and thoughts and a need to collect myself and tell her the good news.

"Doc," I began to say as the tears built up again.

"Just tell me, Tom."

"I am going back to work."

REFLECTION

"Thank you. Thank you for being inquisitive, for asking questions, for making me want to think more deeply about X, Y, and Z. I am so grateful."

This message came from a colleague (a leader at another healthcare organization) a few years back and it told me far more about my colleague than it ever did about me.

This leader showed gratitude and vulnerability. She led with an open mind and heart, and based on the content of our discussion, lived the traits of a servant leader–the exact opposite of an egocentric leader.

(And that is exactly what we need to truly adapt, innovate, and improve the healthcare system to better serve our patients, families and communities.)

Once I hung up the phone, I sat back, looked up, and gave thanks for leaders such as this: Leaders who are not so set in their ways, not so stuck in their own dogma or their own ego that they are open to considering new ways, new perspectives, new options, all in an effort to better their organization and those they serve.

> *"[C]ontrary to the myth of the 'all-knowing-all-powerful' leader, inspired leadership requires vulnerability: Do we have the courage to show up, be seen, take risks, ask for help, own our mistakes, learn from failure, lean into joy, and can we support the people around us in doing the same?"* -- Brené Brown shared in the post *"Leadership Series: Vulnerability and Inspired Leadership.*

Now, perhaps it was the time of year (Thanksgiving), but my conversation above was linked to some sad news that actually led to a place of gratitude and then (the beginning of a New Year) a vision for a new beginning.

In following up this conversation, I reached out to my contact at the Joint Commission to schedule another call and learned that Jerod Loeb, M.D., executive vice president of Healthcare Quality and Evaluation at the Joint Commission, [whose wife Sherri Loeb (a wonderful nurse) is also another amazing servant leader] had passed away after courageously battling cancer for two years.

Jerod was another extraordinary, brilliant, servant leader. He used his own experiences as a patient to further improve the quality of care provision. He focused on improving patient *safety, set a vision for creating high reliability organizations (HROs) and much more. I was blessed to have spoken with Jerod and his team on a few occasions (and to have read much of his work), noting every experience as inspiring.*

The U.S. healthcare system is profoundly broken and sorely needs the type of leader each of us can and should embody. People like my colleague and Jerod Loeb.

These are the types of leaders we need to shift the paradigm from a healthcare to a healthCARING system. These are the types of leaders I hope to be.

Questions

1. As a healthcare leader, when was the last time you were courageous?
    a. When was the last time you were vulnerable and shared this vulnerability with your team or family?
    b. When was the last time your team or family saw your authentic self?
    c. How have you celebrated your failures (as a colleague calls it "failing forward")? How have you grown, learned and improved yourself?
    d. How have you taken risks in order to benefit those you are blessed to serve?
2. As a healthcare leader or clinician, when was the last time you leaned into joy and brought joy to all those around you?
    a. How have you led, served and supported others to do the same?
    b. When was the last time you truly inspired others to achieve a goal or mission and to serve others with care, compassion and love?

Chapter 48

Back to Work

Early the following Monday morning, and for the first time in many many months, I drove myself to the office, this time to a new office in the same building as Saul, arriving before 8:00am.

"Good morning, Adelle. How are you today?"

Adelle was Saul's Executive Assistant.

"Tom! You are back. We missed you! I am so happy you are better. We all are."

It felt so good to be back. And it felt so good to be welcomed back in such a caring way.

"Adelle, I am going to get a cup of coffee and then try to find my new office," I said half kiddingly as I put my briefcase down just outside the kitchen.

"Coffee is all set and I believe your office is upstairs."

Upstairs?

After fixing myself a cup, I walked to the stairway leading to the second floor and grabbed the banister (while looking around to make sure no one was looking).

Coaching myself, *You can do this, Tom,* I slowly began the ascent.

There must have been a dozen steps, but I made it. *Check!*

Arriving on the landing of the second floor, I looked around and saw Robert Johnson from the finance team just coming out of his shared office.

"Tom! You are back! Welcome! Welcome to 'Chez Admin'! I bet you are looking for your office."

Got to love finance folks. Always right to the point.

"Hi Robert. Great to see you and great to be back," I said while again trying to hide the fact that I was gasping a bit for air. "And yes, helping me find my office would be great."

"No problem, Tom. You are on the third floor. The only one up there."

Third floor?

I walked toward the front of the building and turned to my left. Here I found a closed door in a location which would only make sense to open to a closet or to another staircase.

And as I opened the door and saw the albicant stairway rising before me, my mind flashed back to the darkness and murk of my recent nightmares … and I shuddered.

The darkness where people were being hurt each and every day within the healthcare system. The murk creating barriers to navigating the system. The darkness of people harming and being harmed because the system is so broken, and the murk of the aloneness built into the system for clinicians and patients and families alike.

And as I continued to look up with my heart pounding and my breath shallow, I thought about the many flames of goodness within the broken healthcare system as well … like the Mikes in transport and the Lindas, my nurses, and how each kept me safe and cared about me. I thought about Saul and all he is doing to improve the system. I thought about all the wonderful and amazing people I had been blessed to work with to try to make things better. I thought about Tory and Mandy, two incredible and caring nurses, who quite probably saved my life. And I thought about Ben and the model of healthcare he was practicing and how without him I truly believe I would still be wallowing in and out of the broken system, which had given up on me … or worse.

Yes, I continued to have thoughts about the goodness and the brokenness of the healthcare system, and about all I didn't know I didn't know until now, while also understanding there is still much for me to learn.

I thought about my wife and kids, I thought about my team and our mission, I thought about relationships and trust … I thought about love.

I thought about Mrs. Jones (who did so remind me of my Nana) and Mrs. Jones' husband, and I thought about how she represents so many patients we were not listening to, we were not honoring, we were not keeping safe, and we were harming.

And as I continued to look up at the steep staircase before me, truly beginning to understand the depths of the ascent, I took a deep breath and said with all I had and with all my heart …

"We got this."

GAME ON!

REFLECTION

Imagine managing a significant health challenge and needing professional help.

Take a moment and visualize not knowing where to turn or what to do next...

Over time, you learn that you can go online to a website and see which medical school a physician has attended, whether or not the physician is licensed in your state, and their specialty.

Your friends have told you about another website where you can assess the quality of physicians and see the number of blue ribbons they have received.

You follow your friends' recommendations. You identify a physician who is clearly an expert in her field. She is licensed and certified in your state. She has graduated from one of the best medical schools in the country. She has received a number of blue ribbons for clinical guideline adherence.

You make your selection and are comforted by these data. You are in good hands.

You visit this new physician and within 7 minutes you have your diagnosis and are off to pick up your prescription (as per the clinical guidelines).

While at the pharmacy, you access your iPad tablet. You GOOGLE your new diagnosis and in so doing begin to follow a variety of interesting links.

You go to the NPR website and find an interview with Shannon Brownlee (author of "Overtreated") where you read, "But an enormous amount of medicine is not based in science. In fact, the Institute of Medicine estimates that maybe half of what physicians do has valid evidence to back it up. And David Eddy, MD, an expert in medical evidence, says he thinks it's about 15 percent."

Intrigued, you continue your search and see that according to a study published in the Archives of Internal Medicine and referenced by Douglas Perednia, MD, in his blog post "only 14% of the 4,218 individual recommendations (from 41 clinical guidelines) released by the Infectious Diseases Society of America between 1994 and 2010 were based upon properly randomized controlled trials."

After becoming a little discouraged, you decide to relax and read THE ATLANTIC *when you come across the article "Lies, Damned Lies, and Medical Science." From this article, you see that Dr. John Ioannidis and his team have determined that between a third and a half of the most acclaimed research in medicine have been proven to be untrustworthy.*

Lastly you turn to the New Yorker *and you find "The Truth Wears Off" article and begin to read about the "decline effect" and its application to clinical research outcomes and you begin to further understand the challenges of empiricism.*

Processing all of this information, you refer back to the blue ribbons awarded to your new physician for clinical guideline adherence and you hope that the guidelines she (and now you) are following were derived from the research that IS considered trustworthy, from the properly randomized controlled trials and where the decline effect has not been shown to be in play.

You begin to wonder how even the best of the best clinical guidelines that are resultant from the trustworthy research and properly randomized controlled trials can be effective for each and every patient. You ask "Are all diabetic patients the same? Are all patients with high blood pressure the same? Am I the same as every other patient with my same diagnosis?"

You think about one of your friends who has the same diagnosis as you and yet who is unfortunately quite overweight, eats a diet high in saturated fats along with lots of carbs, is going through a messy divorce, is dealing with significant financial issues, and is at least ten years older than you.

You consider your own situation. One of your grandparents and two of your cousins have received the same diagnosis as you and your friend. You have two children in college and are taking care of your elderly mother while working fulltime. Your allergies are working overtime, and your gut is just not quite right.

You wonder if a 7-minute office visit with your new physician truly positioned you both to account for all of these variables. And were all of these data points best leveraged in planning your specific course of treatment.

You further contemplate whether the clinical guidelines recommended by your physician are really appropriate for both you and your friend or even for either of you? Or worse could they be harmful?

You reach back out to your new doctor's office to schedule a virtual visit as soon as possible to discuss this newly acquired information.

Then you decide to download a new app for your smart phone a friend told you about to track your nutrition and exercise; and then another which includes guided meditation.

And as you are doing all these things …

You begin to imagine an improved model of healthcare that would better meet your needs, the needs of your family, and the needs of your community.

Questions

1. What does this new model of healthcare look like?
2. As a healthcare leader, please share your story.
3. As a physician, please share your story.
4. As a nurse, please share your story.
5. As a patient, please share your story.
6. As a family member, please share your story.

And together let's make a difference.

Afterword

"Tom, you are not getting off that easy."

It was 1987, and I had just shared with the group a story of my Pa (my grandfather Joe Cary), who had recently passed way.

And as my professor Warren Dahlin hugged me, he continued, "You not only touched me Tom, you touched our entire class."

The class, Death and Dying.

"It took courage this day for you to share what you did. And even more so, how you did. We felt (we feel) what you felt, what you feel. You provoked empathy in 12 minutes for a person none of us knew … and you made us care."

Of course, now even more tears were flowing down my cheeks.

"You reminded us all that getting a healthcare administration degree here at Stonehill College is more than payment models, mitigating risk, funds flow, or even patient flow. It is also about compassion, understanding, connecting, trusting, and caring."

Professor Dahlin was now looking intently into my eyes as he placed his hand on my shoulder and squeezed.

"And you reminded us that while we must focus on patient healing journeys in healthcare, we must also focus on a patient's dying journey (and their family's journey at the same time) … and often it is this final journey that will require all of our humanity to honor all of their humanity. The way you did today for your Pa."

I think of this now, a number of months into the COVID-19 pandemic, as I process the wide variety of impacts this challenge has and will continue to have on healthcare, on patients and families, on doctors and nurses and all who work in healthcare, on communities, and well beyond.

I think of this now, as together we seek a pathway forward to healthCARING, informed by all we learn as we, with the best intentions, make decisions that ideally do great good but possibly do great harm.

In July 2016, as one of eighteen experts, I was asked to predict how technology will transform healthcare. My response:

> *"There is a very important place for technology in the future of healthcare… when incorporated mindfully. When technology becomes the 'solution' doctors and nurses and patients and families get lost in it, and great harm is likely. When technology is incorporated as part of a co-created care path and with the intention to enhance and improve access and the relationship between patients, families and clinicians, each stakeholder will be honored and whole, and the technological tool will be best aligned to support the healing journey."*

And today, as I read headlines such as, "Digital health stocks are surging because 'suddenly now we're in the future,'" I think of the wisdom of Michael S. Klinkman, MD, MS, a physician leader who also works on the frontlines of healthcare during this pandemic:

> *"Only a small fraction of the patients I'm most concerned about can manage video visits. Thursday, I had thirteen virtual patients scheduled, and 11 of these ended up being phone visits, not video. Three of these people had urgent needs for social services or were in severe financial distress and our social work support system is overwhelmed. If nothing else, this crisis has demonstrated that disparities have real consequences."*

Technology and its impacts are great. And yes, we must continue to improve the healthcare system in which we implement this technology to achieve the positive impacts. We must train and coach and provide feedback to doctors and nurses and all who will be engaging within the system in this new way. And teach them to connect humanely through the process. To connect at the heart, mind, and spiritual level even if through a channel of wires. And then position them to do so in a way so that they too maintain their humanity in the process.

But even that is not enough.

We must also ensure that those who are most vulnerable are also well-positioned to engage in this new way, and if that is not possible, that other paths exist to ensure that they too receive the care they need. The care they deserve. The most vulnerable among us deserve more than an electronic transactional interface. In fact, we all do.

And we must ensure that the human connection, where relationship and trust lead to truth and a pathway forward to address social determinants (influencers) of health together with patients and families, is not overshadowed by the technology associated with screening, identifying, referring, and tracking of the needs.

We must ensure we invest as much (if not more) in human connection and the social, mental health, and other medical and non-medical services themselves as we do in the technology of the process. All important. Humanity most important.

Technology must be incorporated to enhance and improve relationship, not replace it.

Abraham Verghese, MD, in his TED Talk "A Doctor's Touch" coins the term the *iPatient* based on our already (pre-pandemic) overreliance on technology at the expense of the real patient.

"I joke, but I only half joke, that if you come to one of our hospitals missing a limb, no one will believe you till they get a CAT scan, MRI, or orthopedic consult."

Such a poignant warning as the pandemic is driving us more and more toward technology as a solution rather than as a tool.

And it is here as well that Verghese introduces us to a truly transformational opportunity in healthcare:

"I'd like to introduce you to the most important innovation I think in medicine to come in the next ten years, and that is the power of the human hand: to touch, to comfort, to diagnose, and to bring about treatment."

As we seek additional opportunities to keep our patients and families, our clinical team, and our communities safe, we must be mindful (and heartful) that the pendulum doesn't swing too far and we lose the true purpose of why we are here. To care for and care about others and to do so with authentic human connection, appropriate caring touch, with compassion for self and others, and with love for all.

Personal protective equipment (PPE) is essential to safety in the healthcare setting and ensuring ample supply and appropriate use is a must. And we must also understand that masks and other safety equipment create additional barriers to human connection, compassion, and trust. Some clinical team members are ensuring they have light-hearted masks that lead to discussion and levity. Others are ensuring pictures of themselves without the masks are prominent on their clothing. Others are using shields which allow the team member's smile to shine through … all while ensuring safety. Yes, PPE is essential. As is creativity and ensuring the humanity of healthcare aka healthCARING is not lost. As leaders, let us learn from our teams.

The pandemic has also led to quarantines as we seek to flatten the curve and keep people safe – a noble and critical goal. However, as with any improvement opportunity, we must measure the intended outcomes (consequences) and those that were not intended (unintended consequences) as we seek to continuously learn and improve. Unintended negative impacts of the quarantine include, for instance, the uptick in domestic violence and child abuse, the growth of food insecurity, and the exacerbation of mental health issues from isolation and loss.

> *"My Auntie Carol has passed away. I am hurting, but even more so my cousins are hurting. They are not allowed to celebrate her life together as a family. To say goodbye. To hold one another. Closure. The damage to them is immense, and the resources they need are not available…"*

> *"Faith's favorite Uncle was placed in a nursing home and there he unfortunately caught the coronavirus. He died yesterday … isolated. Faith was not allowed to be with him during his final moments on this earth. He died scared and so very alone. She is devastated. There must be a better way."*

We must do better and utilize quality improvement principles and appropriate measurement in the process to ensure that we are not only aware of the positive impacts but also the negative impacts and communicating (informing) transparently and while continuously addressing holistically for the betterment of all.

The pandemic has also highlighted even more so the health inequities and racial disparities within our existing healthcare system. Our most vulnerable continue to be adversely impacted by the system we have created and are being harmed each and every day. Communities of color are being hit disproportionately hard by COVID-19.

"I think it's incumbent on all of us to realize that the health of all of us depends on the health of each of us," says Dr. Alicia Fernandez, a professor of medicine at the University of California San Francisco, whose research focuses on health care disparities.

And as noted by Maria Godoy and Daniel Wood in their piece for National Public Radio (npr), "What Do Coronavirus Racial Disparities Look Like By State":

- Nationally, African American deaths from COVID-19 are nearly two times greater than would be expected based on their share of the population. In four states, the rate is three or more times greater.
- In 42 states plus Washington D.C., Hispanics/Latinos make up a greater share of confirmed cases than their share of the population. In eight states, it's more than four times greater.

This is a wakeup call that should not have been necessary. This is a call to action that is far too late. We must act and we must positively impact now. There is no tomorrow for many members of our community.

As leaders we must use a multi-lens approach when making decisions. We must understand the intended and the unintended consequences. We must own our decisions and when we realize the impact of a decision is bad, we must look in the mirror and we must change.

> *Integrity is doing the right thing when it is unpopular, when everyone is looking, and it places you at risk. Integrity is making the necessary changes for betterment even when it means you must admit to yourself and others that you were wrong.*

The pandemic is teaching us much each and every day. Only with heart and mind wisdom, integrity, togetherness, and right-action will we not only survive, but thrive.

And as we follow this pathway forward, we must honor all those we have harmed by learning from our mistakes and carrying our message forward in word and in deed:

> *Never again shall we harm. Never again shall we sacrifice our most vulnerable. Never again shall we economize compassion, goodness, kindness, empathy, caring. Never again shall profit margin, market share, legacy, ego, or fear overrule integrity, love, and caring. Never again shall we shy away from the tough decisions. Never again shall we hide from truth. Never again shall we hurt another. Not on our watch. Never again.*

Acknowledgements

I love book acknowledgements. As I read them, I make note of the vast numbers of people who contribute to creating and delivering a message. I also relish the gratitude and as we know gratitude heals in and of itself.

Thank you to my bride, Darlene aka Doc. Her power animal is the black bear and she embodies this power as she cares for me, our children, our critters, and all she loves. Without Doc's love, support, wisdom and guidance this work of heart would not exist.

To my daughter Samantha. Sammy shows courage, strength and resiliency each day as she puts herself out to the universe openly and oh so impactfully. And through her own company Dahlborg Designs, produces all the graphic designs for each of my books. I am so proud and thankful.

To my son, Tommy. Without his courage, strength, vulnerability, passion and caring for his friends and family, I would not have learned and grown as a leader and as a person. His podcast Strength thru Vulnerability touches lives and saves souls. I am awed by the man he is.

To my daughter Haylee. Albeit the slightest in physical stature and the youngest in our family, Haylee is mentally strong and someone who will not be denied. She has a spirit which sores and I know will lead her to fly to grand destinations of adventure. She is tough minded and yet so caring and supportive. She loves and cares about this planet and the most vulnerable and throughout her life will educate and impact many.

To my beloved pup, Gabriel. Always there by my side as I write. And always there each evening when I arrive home after a tough day. Not judging. Just loving.

My good friend Rachel Riverwood is my truth. When I write, and it is lousy, she tells me. And she does so with kindness and compassion. She is a true friend who I respect and adore.

Kay Kendall is an impactful leader. She has been a key supporter throughout each of my writing journeys. She is an advisor, a confidant, an editor but most importantly a friend.

Kristin Walker defines the term genuine. Kristin, through her Mental Health News Radio Network and through her friendship, has inspired many a deep discussion relative to mental health, healthcare, leadership, courage, vulnerability, authenticity and much more.

I have been blessed to work with many brilliant leaders, known for their integrity and heart and how they position individuals and teams for optimal impact. People like Jack O'Connor and Paul Hart Miller at Harvard Community Health Plan, Susan Hunt at Beech Street, RaNae Wright at Studer Group, and so many others. Their leadership has informed who I am and how I lead.

To Craig Higgins, PhD, and Warren Dahlin, MS. Two amazing professors at Stonehill College. Craig taught me how to lead and Warren taught me how to live.

I was also blessed to learn from many amazing physician leaders who combine their leadership skills and clinical wisdom with a keen focus on ensuring patients receive the highest quality care every time. People like Bethany Hays, MD, at the Hygeia Foundation, Charlie Homer, MD, at the National Institute for Children's Health Quality (NICHQ), Alan Kornberg, MD, at Network Health Corporation, Michael S. Klinkman, MD, MS, at the University of Michigan Department of Family Medicine, and David Howes, MD, at Martin's Point Health Care. You each have made a difference in the lives of many.

To the amazing nurse leaders I was blessed to work with and also learn from. People like my bride Darlene Dahlborg, RN, at Harvard Community Health Plan – Staff Model division, Jean Davila, RN, MSN and Laura Malone, RN, BSN, MPA, each at Studer Group, Jennifer Bowe, RN, MSN, RNC, at St. Vincent Medical Center, Vikki Choate, RN, MSN, at Martin's Point Health Care, Ellen Smith Hedger, LVN, and former host of the Chatterbox with Ellen Hedger, and so many others. You each have showed me in action what healthCARING should be and could be.

Greg Thompson, DO, epitomizes the term *healer*. Greg connected with Doc and I at every level. At the heart, mind and soul level. He was caring and loving. Brilliant and dedicated. And he saved my life. I will never forget you.

To Faith. My bride's best friend who supported Doc and was always there for her and for our family when I was sick. Faith is one of those Angel's on earth ... and her name is so very fitting.

To my Dad and Mom. You continue to teach me daily. You have always supported and encouraged me. You made me who I am, and I love you.

My brother Jon. Although physically we are apart, aside from my bride, you are my best friend.

My sister Darlene. You are a dedicated and skilled nurse who shows up each day and ensures your patients are always safe. Thank you.

To all of you on the front lines of healthcare, the Mikes and the Lindas who care and love each patient and family and do so in word and in action. To the engineer at the VA who shared his heart and sought help for his soul. To the housekeepers who keep us all safe. To you all … it is you who are the foundation of a healthCARING system. And it is the rest of us who are grateful.

And to all the patients and families who experience the healthcare system. Thank you for trusting us. I know we have not always earned your trust, but please know we will never stop trying.

To all the readers of this book, thank you for taking the time to read these words, to process these messages, to share your feedback and to each day seek ways to make a difference. We will transform healthcare and we will do so together. May God Bless Each of You.

The Dove

The shivering is constant. The permafrost tearing deep into my soul.

"So cold," I think, "So dark. Why so dark?"

The pressure of the deep makes it impossible to catch my breath.

My ears are completely blocked from the tide's density and barely audible turbulence.

The frigid ocean surrounds me on all sides now as I continue to sink into the black expanse.

"My head, my chest, bursting ... they are going to burst!" I scream into the gloom. "Please God. Please. No mas!"

"Breathe. Breathe," reverberates from the remoteness as my efforts falter and a burden intensifies.

The darkness, the coldness, the pressure. My body acknowledges each as my cells are vised and deserted, I descend into its depths.

"I am afraid, God. Very afraid. Please ..."

My descent continues into perpetuity with all of my emotional nakedness strewn into the eternal darkness.

"No. No. My heart is breaking but it is not broke!" I scream into the nothingness.

"I am not alone! I am not!" I cry into the disquietude.

"Breathe. Breathe." I feel in my core from this struggle in the abyss.

"I am not alone! I don't have to be. I don't need to be! I don't want to be!" I fight as the reality of submersion comes to light and a lightness appears above.

A light? But wait ...

Juxtaposed to the light above remains the mass of shadow being swallowed into an oblivion.

And yet ... and yet, I watch as it departs from me. Slowly. Ever so slowly. But definitely separate from me now. And descending deeper and deeper into the gloom.

The sun is high in the sky casting a gleam over the cove. The leaves on the trees just beyond the marsh are exquisite with fiery reds, deep oranges, and bright yellows. The marshlands themselves almost pink as they glow in the sunlight.

The beam of light burns at my skin and scorpions my eyes as I squint to see the blue green water flowing before me.

I squat in the sand and continue to peer down at the black mass which has left my humanity and is now following its own solo journey into the Sheol of the cove depths.

"We are connected," I hear in the deepness of my Soul as I look beyond myself into the vastness of God's creation. "We are all connected. The Darkness and the Light. Complex. Ever adapting. Connected."

But now, at this moment my darkness is no longer within me but sinking beyond as suddenly the surface of the water is disrupted and a Loon breaks through and flies into the light of the clear blue sky.

"So beautiful," I am saying to no one in particular when I realize this beautiful creature is actually not a Loon. "But it must be. What else can it be?"

I squint my eyes even tighter as the light of the sun continues to shine.

"If not a Loon ... then it must be ..."

I continue to breathe and squint and squint and breathe as finally this flying creature comes into focus and I realize it is truly not a Loon. But rather ...

… a Dove.

"A dove has escaped the murk and the depths," I say out loud. "A dove is no longer alone in the dark and the cold. A dove is now flying into the infinity before it. A dove is now soaring beyond its perceived limits. A dove is seeking its partner, its place. A dove is no longer alone."

"It is a dove. It is not a loon. It is a dove." I scream at the top of my lungs as joy overtakes me.

"A dove! It is saved, my Love! I am saved. Never to be alone again."

Disruption

crisis affecting all
no one left out
hurting hearts
spirits crushed
loneliness abounds
fear new and constant
accelerated change
toughened resolve
stronger commitment
kindness abounds
resilience
love

- Jennifer Bowe, Frontline nurse leader

BONUS MATERIAL

The Gilded Age of Healthcare

Some years back, my family and I visited a plethora of colleges in Rhode Island as my oldest daughter sought her life's path. On our way from Bristol to Newport I shared with my family my days of working for Harvard Community Health Plan (before it became Harvard Pilgrim Health Care) in that area and the large disparity between the wealthiest and the poorest (primarily people of color) in Newport at that time (mid-1990s).

After a brief tête-à-tête, my bride and I agreed to take a slight excursion from the college tours and visit two of "the Mansions" in Newport, the Breakers and Marble House.

As we began the self-guided audio tour, I was again thinking about the wealth disparity back in the 1990s and how large the disparity must have been in the 1880s, when these homes were built. And just as I started to process how conceptually things have not changed, I heard in my ears (via the self-guided tour) the words of Mark Twain's "The Gilded Age." The gilded age I thought. "The golden gleam of the gilded surface hides the cheapness of the metal underneath."

I turned to my bride and I shared what I was thinking: "These Mansions–the gilded age– remember that piece I wrote some months back about "bricks and mortar" and how the construction of these new hospitals and hospital wings and extravagant new medical office buildings serve to 'represent power, conquest, legacy building, and achievement, and yet are not always in line with what is best for the populace?' The mansions and their gilded surfaces served the same purpose."

As I continued to think about the wealth disparity when these mansions were built, my mind drifted to the poor who currently line up outside of the local new and/or expanded hospital hoping for someone to show compassion, to care, to empathize, to help.

I further contemplated Twain's quote, "the gilded surface hides the cheapness of the metal underneath," and reflected back on the hospital leaders who built these shiny new palaces of which 69 percent do not deem quality and patient safety as top priorities. An example of Twain's "underneath"?

I thought about the physicians who are working in these gorgeous new medical office buildings and yet are subjected to intense productivity quotas (like factory workers) and do not have time to know their patients, develop trust with their patients, share empathy with their patients, and co-create patient-specific care plans that address the root-cause of their health challenges.

I considered the financing of healthcare within these dazzling facilities and how overtreatment is rewarded and yet is also placing patients in harm's way.

My thoughts turned to the gilded "patient-centered" concept being lauded, and I wondered how can care be patient centered if…

… the physician does not have the time to know the patient?
… the bottom line is more important than the patient?
… the system does not care enough to have accurate medical information available to the physician and patient at time of service?

Perhaps all of this patient-centered languaging is the "gild" and the reality of patient-centered care is the "cheapness of the metal underneath."

Despite wealth disparity, we continue to see these gilded hospital systems and health care practices but witness less and less focus on effectively addressing the needs (physical, mental, emotional, cultural, environmental, financial, etc. aka Social Determinants (Influencers) of Health) of our most vulnerable populations.

Is it really too quixotic to want the "underneath" in healthcare to match the "gild"?

I don't believe so.

We are talking about the health of our friends, our families, and our communities. Beautiful mansions like the stunning new hospitals, spectacular hospital wings, and mighty medical complexes are only as gilded as the hope, the provision, the safety, the outcomes, the care and the caring, and the service they provide to patients and families.

Looking beyond the gild, we have much work to do. And together we will ensure the golden gleam and gild on the surface of healthcare runs deep within the hearts of all healthcare leaders and thus all healthcare systems.

For it is only with the engaged heart of leadership partnering with those who need us most we will finally close the gap of disparity and inequity and injustice for all.

Cultural Competence is a Leadership Choice
The Seven Steps

As a leader here are seven steps you can take today to not only improve cultural competence within your organization, but also the health of your organization, the health of your team, and the health of your community:

1. Set a clear vision for care and identify cultural competence as a priority. Learn about your community, their cultural backgrounds, their traditions and where they seek care. Identify disparities and act to close the gap. Go beyond collecting market data. Rather, become part of the community by engaging and serving all members. As an example, many hospitals have partnered with faith-based institutions to broaden their reach in the community.

2. Build a culturally competent care model that meets the needs of the entire community. Invest, embrace, and honor the mosaic of your community. If your community has a large non-English speaking population, communicate with this group using their native language. If traditional healing makes sense for your community, engage traditional healers. If members of your community do not seek care within the four walls of your hospital, then go to them. Some years ago, in Chicago, access was improved dramatically when care was provided in a barbershop, a favorite gathering place for African American males in that area. It was an innovative and engaging program to meet people where they are. Learn from innovations in other communities and then do so similarly.

3. Be aware of power differentials that can create distrust for the medical community. The majority of doctors in the United States are male, white and affluent – but many patients are not. Some patients may hesitate to seek care because of this disparity. Also, when these same patients choose to see a provider, they may feel anxious about discussing their health and lifestyle for fear of being judged or misunderstood. When providers promote an open, non-judgmental atmosphere, it encourages patients to communicate freely, leading to optimal care.

4. Meet patients where they are and not where we want them to be. Take the time to learn about the patient's and family's culture, and don't assume everyone from the same culture has the same belief system. Recognize that there is a cultural connection between physical, mental, emotional and spiritual health. Be open to understanding healing and dying preferences, and work with the patient and family to integrate these choices into their overall care plan.

5. Listen carefully to patients. Dr. William Osler once said, "Listen to your patient; he is telling you the diagnosis." As humans, we are programmed to listen to respond. The real impact is when we listen to understand. To do so, we must expand our view, focus on establishing a connection with each patient and family and be open to learning new approaches that are also safe and effective.

6. Create more ways for diverse members of your community to become part of your institution's workforce. To open your employee pipeline, consider networking with diverse professional and alumni associations, advertising in culturally appropriate media outlets and partnering with universities, community colleges and high schools.

7. Develop Patient and Family Advisory Councils (PFACs) to actively engage diverse members of your community and do so with a commitment to leverage their wisdom. This must not be a "check the box" activity but an authentic relationship built on trust as part of the organization's strategy to reach everyone. And within this forum collaboratively develop the systems, structures and processes that support equity and prioritize and address the social determinants (influencers) of health impacting the most vulnerable in your community.

The goal is to improve care and outcomes for everyone.

To do so we must embrace diversity by honoring and respecting all cultures. When each member of our healthcare team delivers culturally competent care, we can profoundly improve safety, quality, and access for all.

And together we will.

Hope Is Not A Strategy
It Is More Important

Many terrific leaders I know often say, "Hope is not a strategy." And for many in healthcare — a world often led by science, evidence and action — many believe this makes a lot of sense. It is logical. And as a terrific physician leader said to me one day, "One cannot just hope for a bus to arrive. Sometimes one must chase after that bus."

That said, my philosophy had always been, "Hope may not be a strategy … but it is even more important. Hope is the foundation for All."

Hope is what gets many people up in the morning — especially in healthcare and especially during times of crisis (think COVID-19).

We are moved to act by the Hope that we will make a difference.

We act decisively with the firm Hope that we will make things better.

We push ourselves beyond our limits enlivened by the Hope that we will save a life … a soul … a community.

Without Hope it doesn't matter if we have the soundest strategy.

Without Hope people won't be present, people won't be inspired, people will not take the right action when times are tough, and we will not achieve betterment for others.

That said, my thinking has evolved as of late.

When we bring Hope together with Faith — we instill Courage (the root word for courage is *couer*, meaning heart) — and we move into right action.

And here is why…

At the heart of Faith is conviction. It is an inherent truth we feel in our hearts and in our souls. It is an innate belief that even if something seems to make no sense cognitively, with Faith and Hope and Courage we will proceed to transcend the hopeless, we impact, and make a difference for others.

Hopelessness leads to the inaction of despondency and doubt. When we think things are truly hopeless, we do not act – because no specific action makes any sense. Hope and Faith leads to acts of inner strength against the hopelessness of stagnation and with Courage in the mix overcomes paralyzing fear.

Sometimes Faith and Hope are all we have, and as leaders and as people on the front lines of healthcare, we must leverage each to inspire our teams, our patients and their families, and our communities who are often scared, who are hurting, who truly need us.

One morning while sitting in the lobby of a V.A. hospital I heard, "Guess what I have in the box."

This veteran and I had been conversing for the past twenty minutes. He noticed my Boston accent immediately. And I noticed his Brooklyn. (We were neither in Boston nor Brooklyn).

"I have an angel in this box."

He had told me about his branch. His service. His war. He said he loves the V.A. He said he loves seeing his brothers and sisters here. He said he misses his wife (who he had lost a few years back to cancer.)

"Why do you have an angel in a box?"

My new friend was quiet for a moment.

"I recently had surgery here."

He proceeded to tell me the details. How he did not want the surgery. How cold the operating room was. How they had trouble waking him in recovery.

As he spoke the lobby became more and more busy. I lean forward and continue to listen.

"I have seen a lot. I have done a lot. I don't like to admit it, but I was really scared. Mary [his wife] was no longer here keeping me safe."

He continued.

"And I kept having bad memories of losing my Mary."

He began to weep.

"I am so sorry."

We waited. The lobby became silent (at least to us) as our safe space was held. He took a deep breath. I noticed I was holding mine.

"Why do you have an angel in a box?"

More silence. More shared space holding.

"I was so scared. I want to be with Mary. I really do. I miss her so."

Silence.

"But I also know I have more to do here."

I remember to breathe.

"When I awoke in recovery, as my eyes cleared and the world came back into focus, I saw her. And then I heard her. My nurse. Nurse Michelle."

More silence. More space.

"Master Sargent, Jim … This is Michelle. Your nurse. You are in recovery. You did great. Your surgery is done. You did so good. Jim … "

Silence.

"Tom, Michelle held my hand. She leaned in. She spoke softly. She was so calming. She cared about me. She had Faith. She gave me Hope. … Just like my Mary."

More silence.

"I felt safe. And I believed I would be okay."

We each took a breath.

"Michelle was my angel and I want her to know."

Share Hope. Have Faith. Be Courageous. Then Lead, Serve and Love.

Always. All ways.

Author Bio

With well over thirty-five years of extensive healthcare leadership experience, Tom is a voice for relationship centered and compassionate care, servant leadership and quality and systems improvement.

An author, leader and advisor, he is also an internationally recognized speaker and writer with an expertise in healthCARING models, heart and mind communication, courageous vulnerability, systems thinking and improvement, stopping bullying, adverse childhood experiences (ACES) and bringing "love in action" to all we do.

He is a father, husband and coach. A coach to healthcare leaders. And a coach to young men.

Tom has written the book, *The Big Kid and Basketball ... and the lessons he taught his Father and Coach*, where he shares stories of bullying, resiliency, parenting, coaching, faith, family and love.

He is also a contributor to the book, *Bullied Back to Life*, focusing on how victims of bullying have used their experiences to fuel their success, and how you can too.

And a contributor to the Amazon Best Selling book, *Highway to Heart, Humor, and Honesty in Healthcare*, a book for healthcare providers, patients, and family members who desire to understand how to better connect with one another.

Tom believes at the end of the day it is all about impact.

"What good is it for someone to gain the whole world, yet forfeit their soul?"

- Mark 8:36

Made in the USA
Las Vegas, NV
16 November 2020